The Wounded Physician Project

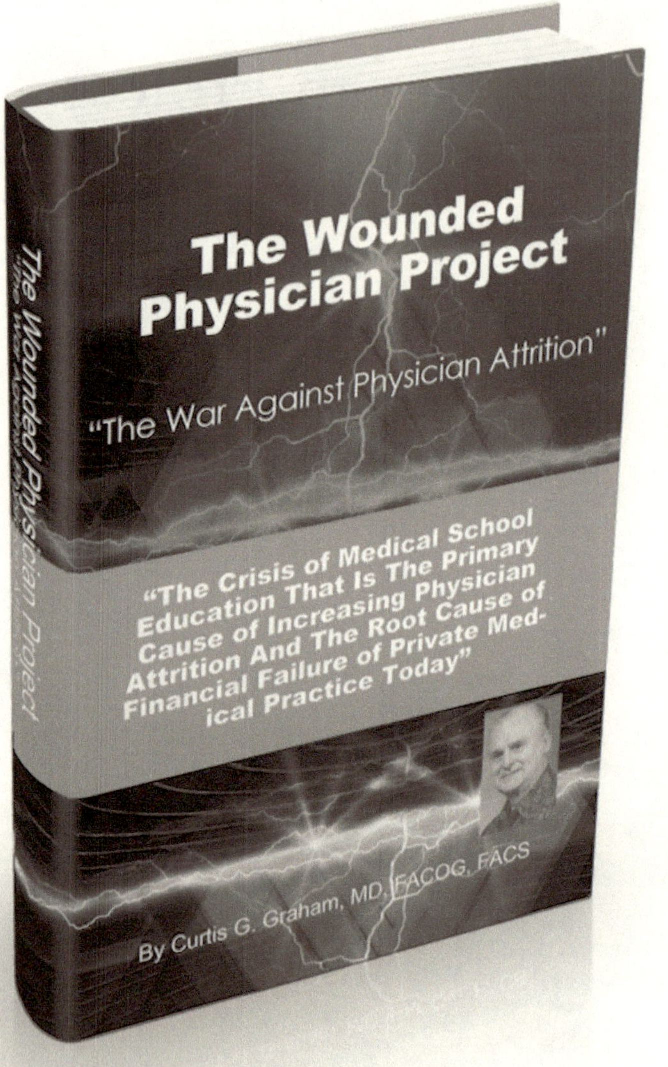
The Wounded Physician Project
"The War Against Physician Attrition"
"The Crisis of Medical School Education That Is The Primary Cause of Increasing Physician Attrition And The Root Cause of Financial Failure of Private Medical Practice Today"
By Curtis G. Graham, MD, FACOG, FACS
The Wounded Physician Project

The Wounded Physician Project

Curtis G. Graham, MD, FACOG, FACS

Library of Congress Control Number:		2014919526
ISBN:	Hardcover	978-1-4990-8338-5
	Softcover	978-1-4990-8339-2
	eBook	978-1-4990-8340-8

This book was printed in the United States of America.

Rev. date: 12/17/2014

To order additional copies of this book, contact:
Xlibris
1-888-795-4274
www.Xlibris.com
Orders@Xlibris.com
663515

CONTENTS

INTRODUCTION

THE THOUGHT THAT every practicing physician in our nation is presently caught in a web of professional and career uncertainty demands an aggressive stance against every threat that seeks to change our professional freedom to that of being an indentured servant (employees).

Increasing and relentless governmental intrusions into medical practice result in the compromise of every doctor's fundamental expectations and aspirations for their career in private medical practice under the guise of improving the availability of healthcare and ultimately reducing the cost of healthcare... which will never happen.

In this treatise you will learn several factors that are the primary causes for the rapidly rising attrition of physicians as well as the grass root causes of their frustrations that lead to their attrition, to which little attention has been paid.

In addition, the problem about who is rightly responsible for the business education of medical doctors is debated.

Many approaches are suggested in this book to solve the issue of the business education of medical students and include reasons why medical schools are the most appropriate place and time for providing this "medical business" education.

Because I have personally experienced every untoward aspect of this treatise during my active military, employed, and private medical practice years, I feel qualified and obligated to offer legitimate and reasonable solutions.

My comments are experience driven, as factual as possible, and speak to the necessary changes that need to be made for the survival of private medical practice as well as the financial survival of all physicians in private medical practice.

"There are four important things that I would like you to keep in mind while reading this book."

1. **I want you to understand the real and actual causes of the problems that are most likely to continue destroying private medical practice that you may have not considered or acted upon.**

Riding the wave of extreme frustration and utter disappointment so widespread among doctors in private practice goes far beyond the usual feelings of frustration commonly experienced in previously normal medical practice. Overwhelming frustration and uncertainty destroys the passion to continue to practice medicine.

Physicians don't really go through the education, training, and practice of medicine for the welfare of our citizens or our healthcare system, contrary to what others may say and think. Desire to help people (medically) drives the passion to become a physician, but it gradually dissipates thereafter.

The firstborn passion after completing medical school and specialty training changes to a passion to provide a well-deserved lifestyle for their family and themselves. Yes, it's a selfish trait. After all, survival is instinctual, especially when we are talking about family.

The essential means of satisfying this passion is to use their medical practice to create an income that will be adequate for reaching their anticipated career goals and family lifestyle obligations.

The tragedy today is that very few physicians ever reach those career or practice goals that they established in their minds at the beginning of medical school.

That happens in private practice today because physicians can't earn enough money to satisfy their ego, passion to excel, family needs and expectations, and their own personal desires.

Sure, they love to practice medicine and to cure illness, but when you *take away the benefits expected* from their medical career, the desire to help the sick and injured takes second place in priority. If that means that it becomes necessary to change careers, most will do it in a split second. A good backup career plan would be smart to have and keep available.

The greatest dilemma that medical school scholars have is to accept the fact that a student's passion to become a physician doesn't continue to exist and keep them in practice after the entire medical educational gauntlet is completed.

There are many more powerful forces that overshadow one's passion to be or to remain a physician once they begin medical practice. Those forces that keep doctors in medical practice are what this book is all about… all related to the business of medical practice.

Anyone who has been in the situation of telling their spouse that there isn't enough money from the medical practice coming in for the kid's college education or to create a reasonable retirement plan understands what I mean.

Relative poverty is not what physicians signed up for, or expected, especially when there's an average of $150,000 educational debt hanging over their heads by graduation time and that is likely to keep them in relative poverty for years to come.

The source of the frustration is lack of adequate money in their pockets. This situation hits home when friends or family are in a commercial business they own and are making two or three times the net income of a doctor who is practicing today.

Doctors have a reason to complain and feel betrayed by the profession, especially when a fast food restaurant manager with a high school education makes more money than many doctors. It's a time when doctors begin to question whether they can do better financially outside of the profession and, actually, they can.

2. **I want you to understand how serious of an issue business education and knowledge is for the whole medical profession in terms you should consider to be *more than urgent.***

There is a way to improve the financial situation and capabilities of every physician in private practice… even those physicians who are employed in the future. When physicians have an *academic business education background* before starting medical practice, they have a tremendous offensive capability to push their medical practice business income far above the usual, do it faster, and do it persistently. Do you doubt that? Maybe you should think about it for a while?

The problem is *that medical schools do not intend to provide a formal business education to medical students* nor do they feel any obligation to do so. The obligation has been shifted to someone else (medical students/doctors). This belief structure is called the "normalcy bias."

***Definition*: Formal or academic business education as related to medical education of physicians.**
It means that the business education is presented to students in a classic, methodical, and instructive teaching format using advanced techniques, tactics, and materials that have the most pronounced, effective, and enduring qualities equal to or surpassing any advanced postgraduate academic course concerning most business principles and practices.

Therefore, medical students are, in reality, being provided with *only half of a full medical "practice" education.* The logic follows that medical schools, by any standard of responsibility in my opinion, are inherently responsible for educating "financially disabled" doctors who will consequently never have the opportunity to reach their maximum potential and productivity during their medical careers. Have you ever considered why so many doctors today might feel betrayed by their medical school?

Anyone who believes that any financially burned-out private practice physician or any graduating medical student will take time away from their medical practice or training to obtain a formal business education they need must also be a senior member of the flat earth society.

How do you set with these issues?

3. **I want you to understand how an academic business education program can be created and implemented into the present four-year standing medical school education curriculum without distracting from the medical education process, and why.**

The creation and implementation of an academic business curriculum can be done by a person or group with an entrepreneurial mindset. It can be done inexpensively and efficiently (compared with other medical school projects).

The leader of this project needs organizational skills, determination, leadership skills, and integrity--a special kind of person. Your know a leader with an overwhelming passion and belief that this project is dictated by the integrity of academic commitment to educate all medical students to meet every challenge (business and medical) they will face in practice.

Such a profound and unique means of establishing a significantly higher standard of professional education of physicians morally exceeds the ability to align the educational objectives with the end users.

Is there any other means to provide this business education at a better time, in a better educational environment, at a time when the mind is best prepared to learn, or at a better available time in a medical student's career program? I haven't found one.

I've included a sample set of details about how this project and its alternatives can be added and implemented to the advantage of all concerned.

4. **I want to convince you of the absolute and desperate necessity for medical education academics to create and provide an academic business education for every medical student.**

Given the present healthcare crisis (2014), there is no better time to stand up for what you believe will sustain the basic foundation of the practice of medicine.

After decades of "prehistoric thinking" within the academic medical education community and their failure to remain in control of our profession, we are left helpless to do much about the external circumstances that enslave us.

The regretful aspect of this new controlling "progressive" governmental initiative is that we now can see our mistake of failing to take protective actions years ago. When the medical education scholars saw, and then ignored, the obvious deficiency (a formal business education) in our medical school education system, we became decisively vulnerable to the whims of politics and politicians.

The deficiency of not providing an academic business education for all medical students over the many decades of unrecognized medical practice mediocrity is an indication that *medical education tradition is the enemy* of common sense and the enemy *regarding maximum potential of physicians.*

It's not that medical education scholars didn't know medical practice is a business and that it requires a significant business education to withstand the assaults from predators and competition, but the fact that they were unable to open their mindsets to solutions that would have made remarkable improvements to the medical profession years ago.

Instead, the medical school academics chose to hide from their obligation to provide for an academic business education by passing that obligation on to the medical students and physicians themselves. We all understand the many customary reasons why they would choose to do that and think that way.

But this inexcusable neglect and results of that neglect are clearly visible over at least the past seven decades of medical practice in our nation. The mistaken belief that medical students predictably would be smart enough, diligent enough, and motivated enough to obtain business education on their own sometime later, has proven to be profoundly wrong.

The sad part is that physicians (with rare exceptions) do not take the time to obtain a formal business education after leaving medical school. But who can blame them for not doing it? Physicians would rather stumble along in their mediocre medical practice business, perpetually making bad business decisions that they don't recognize in the first place as being bad.

And physicians unconsciously accept the unrecognized consequences of "absent" business knowledge and remain "unconscious" of the astounding financial and business problems it creates for them in medical practice. When this all happens unconsciously, they consciously think that they are at the top of their game in medicine--even though they aren't! They believe it because they have never been taught the successful business standards to have a basis for comparison.

That corrupted mindset is the primary source of disaster in private medical practice today!

We've already waited for over fifty years to see who will accept responsibility for *telling physicians and medical students* that a formal business education is critical to maximum medical practice business success. And, who will also guarantee that at least the medical school students get the business education all physicians need today?

Nobody has shown up to accept the challenge!

Now, do we forget the obligation stuff and let fate become the mediator of our careers? Looks like it to me. And that's one of my reasons for shouting out about the importance of implementing this undertaking of a business education for all medical students.

You will find in this book the details of what can be done to resolve this issue as well as the benefits to everyone (students, doctors, patients, medical profession) involved in the undertaking.

"In a gentle way you can shake the world." -Mahatma Gandhi

It disturbs me deeply that there has been what seems to be a consensus of opinion among medical education scholars and expert authorities that the "business of medical practice" should be relegated to the position of professional apostasy.

The history of widespread financial failures of private medical practice continues to expose our professional business education vulnerabilities and ignorance.

Responsibility for providing a formal business education is something that needs to be brought out of the dusty archives of medicine and treated with the respect and discernment that it deserves.

The ongoing enigma about the "medical school education" academics refusing to acknowledge this obligation is more than shameful. It's something that today has become the cause for the deterioration of the medical profession rather than its improvement.

Another factor that seems so outrageous and difficult to justify for many of us is the extraordinary effort being made by most medical schools to jam as much medical knowledge as possible into the minds of medical students when large amounts of that medical education will have very little value or use for those physicians later in their careers.

Knowing what I know today, trading all those hours and days learning and being exposed to that "rarely –needed" medical knowledge and replacing that time and energy with a business education would be a hundred times more beneficial to any doctor in medical practice today.

Medical knowledge and skills are primarily only useful in medicine. Business knowledge and skills can be used anywhere, anytime, in any endeavor throughout life. You tell me what's more valuable than this.

These issues are discussed in detail in this book.

PREFACE

NEVER BEFORE IN history has the private practice of medicine been subjected to such devastating and restrictive challenges that now threaten the very freedom of its existence and its survival as a independent medical profession model.

The commoditization of physicians has become a political precedent for our government's manipulation and power building progressive agenda. This has now irreversibly changed the capacity of the medical profession to defend itself.

The freedoms inherent to the delivery of healthcare to medical patients from its most advantageous position and function are being egregiously and increasingly compromised.

However, as constrained as the medical profession currently is, there are many remaining defensive approaches for maintaining elements of the profession that can and will enable the persistence of a number of foundational elements of the profession. The secret is that there are "offensive" tactics as well.

Every physician is well aware of what is happening and would like to preserve their freedom to practice medicine as much as possible independent of increasing governmental interference and control.

The mass exodus of physicians from the profession is something that is suspiciously overlooked, disregarded, and intentionally neglected by those who could creatively reverse those detrimental changes.

Signs of physicians' disappointment with their careers are everywhere, if one chooses to investigate the cause of the profession-wide attrition of physicians. Feelings of helplessness among physicians to be able to do anything to prevent or reduce the takeover of the medical profession are widespread for good reason. Fee restrictions have undoubtedly become the dominant factor that contributes to physician frustration.

It isn't that physicians and medical educators were unaware of the intentions of our government to control healthcare over the last seven decades. It is that organized medicine, sitting in authority, was and is unable to defend against the political system intentions effectively enough to prevent the problems we now face. Enough money, influence, and power have been never enough for organized medicine to overcome the nearly impossible.

How did government slip into this control position?

In the beginning of governmental efforts to control the high costs (promised by the managed care initiatives) of healthcare in about 1970, primarily at the prodding of large union and industrial employers, it seemed like a good idea.

However, physicians were forced to accept the managed care mandates and practice under them. Physicians at that time believed in their own ability to compensate for any fee restrictions and other restrictive issues. This belief, even when they saw large numbers of their own patients move to the PPO's and HMO's, persisted unopposed.

Undoubtedly, all physicians without a business education were left without the *essential business knowledge and tools* to survive financially outside of the managed care mandate. There was no choice but to comply. Even just a basic marketing knowledge would have helped replace the patients who left their private practice.

Many physicians were caught in the trap of agreeing to accept reduced fees to treat those shared medical patients or lose their medical practices. It became a matter of a permanently reduced income for physicians in private practice and much less so for employed physicians.

It was the ideal time for physicians with a business education to use the business tools they had learned to rapidly compensate for their lack of income caused by the managed care mandates.

The problem with that was the fact that 99 percent of medical doctors had no formal business education. Therefore, they learned to compensate somewhat by working harder in practice by trying to increase their patient load... only to end up in practice burn-out.

The impact felt by the physicians

The impact of the lack of a business education over the last seven decades has left physicians running their medical practice businesses with no true knowledge about the time-honored business principles to follow. Of course, employed physicians never had to worry about learning how to run a medical practice business because they have someone else doing it all for them.

The effect of the gradual unnoticed separation of the private and employed medical doctors over the last fifty some years has resulted in a serious and somewhat confrontational division within the medical profession.

Physicians in private practice today continue to suffer not only from the lack of a business education, but also from the lack of support from the seemingly unsympathetic "employed" physicians.

Employed physicians are those who practice in the environment of predictable financial stability and tenure with no true business obligations other than seeing patients, showing up for work, and earning vast amounts of money for the business owners.

Factors that have led to massive physician attrition.

Getting back to the issue of inadequate income, the truth that you can't do much of anything without money, implicates a full set of monetary causes for the frustration and attrition of medical doctors that affect the medical profession today... at least those that are in private medical practice.

If severe frustration and disappointment are found among physicians in at least 50 percent of the private practice physicians as the recent American Medical Association (AMA) survey reveals, there has to be a reason.

The basis for these destructive emotions is no secret. Any physician whose private practice is financially failing and has no capability to reverse the process, will fail.

Physicians with a formal business education to draw from have the tools and strategies to prevent the financial failure to begin with. A business-educated physician is always aware of the factors that indicate when a financial threat is imminent or present and can immediately implement appropriate business tools to bring the practice back on to a successful financial track.

Knowing that over 95 percent of graduating medical students have no sound formal business education instantly forces the question, "How can any private practice medical business today

survive, profit, and grow when it's a business that's run by someone with no business education?"

The real answer comes from the research-based statistics that reveal that 95 percent of small businesses fail in the first five years primarily for the same reason.

No business can survive when the owner of the business doesn't know or use any of the well-known business principles required for business success. The level of success of any business is determined by the effective and productive use of all business tools that are commonly responsible for success.

Applying this to medical practice business means that physicians who have very little business knowledge also should expect very little medical practice financial success.

In business, money is power. The amount of net profits from medical practice provides for the affordable amount of continued education available to any physician as well as the degree of accomplishments and skill sets necessary for reaching every goal that any physician has for his/her career.

The interrelationships that all of the above factors have contributed to a physician's optimal career capabilities and to the physician's maximal attainable potential with the medical practice business are detailed in this book.

"Men are anxious to improve their circumstances
but are unwilling to improve themselves.
They therefore remain bound."
-James Allen, "As a Man Thinketh"

PREMISE

THE PRACTICE OF medicine in all respects is universally accepted to be a professional business when established and managed by independent physicians or managed healthcare systems. Medical practice business is given legal status under the law.

The practice of medicine is universally accepted and understood to be a business entity by every medical educator, medical school, organized medical education system and governing body. It includes those individuals who are specifically tasked with selecting or creating the components of medical education curriculums.

Survival requirements of private medical practice businesses are exactly the same as all successful commercial businesses.

Our professional medical education system is held today to be the *premier medical education system* in the world.

Yet, medical school education scholars in our nation have intentionally disregarded all efforts to provide or arrange for an academic business education for medical students. In spite of the overwhelming proof of and urgent requirement for a business education of physicians (medical students), the medical education hierarchy continues to do nothing to resolve the issue.

Known and accepted throughout the business world for the last century is the fact that business success (for any kind of business) requires special knowledge about managing a business successfully and profitably. That fact, which has been persistently ignored over the past six or seven decades, has contributed a major portion to the cause of the present medical profession crisis.

The deluge of physician attrition and the extreme frustration running rampant throughout private practice of medicine (is at least half of the physician population within our nation) will continue to cause severe problems within the profession unless academic medical scholars take action to fill the void related to the business education of all medical students.

The ease and cost of creating and implementing business education for medical students is neither difficult nor beyond the scope of creative-minded medical educators to provide.

Objective:

A necessary task is the introduction and implementation of a business education curriculum into the four-year medical school curriculum in this world of digital education in every medical school today.

Business education is the most critical factor not only for the financial survival of private medical practice today but also for the retention of physicians in a medical career that they will not be utterly disappointed with.

This mandate for an academic business education being created ASAP for every medical school in our nation will radically improve the business income and productivity of every private practice physician overnight.

For those who envision the future of medical practice as a life of employee servitude to the healthcare bureaucracy already started today, it implies a formidable lack of determination and creativity.

Private medical practice is here to stay. However, the likelihood of the private practice model changing is great. Predictably, the primary model will be some form of concierge or "cash-only" practice. If this becomes a reality, then the importance of an academic business education of medical students will escalate.

With these factors in mind, this mandate is one approach to saving private medical practice and the medical careers of physicians who will otherwise quit or be forced out of medical practice.

"The physician is expected to meet the grim monster, break the jaws of death, And pluck the spoil out of his teeth."

-R. V. Pierce, MD
President, World's Dispensary Medical Association
Buffalo, NY (1895)

MISSION

"This treatise is a universal mandate for final resolution of the unseen financial wounds every physician in private medical practice inevitably sustains in today's world during their private medical practice career."

Primary wounds…

FIRST, *FINANCIAL FAILURE* of medical practices is and has been destroying private medical practice over the last seven decades. *Lack of an academic business education* is the factor that ensures that physicians will never have the business knowledge and tools to recover from financial medical practice difficulties, or to prevent them.

Secondly, because of the lack of a formal business education, all physicians have been and are now being denied *access to the business education essentials* that are required in order for every physician to reach his or her maximum potential in medical knowledge, medical skills, and competence in medical practice. These fatal wounds now account for the probable coming demise of private medical practice.

Cause…

Lack of *academic business education* cripples all private practice physicians' ability to prevent or to overcome the increasing financial stress and inadequate medical practice incomes that are now causing the massive physician attrition from medical practice today.

Solution…

Implementation of an academic business education curriculum during the four-year medical school education process will not only ensure that financial failure doesn't happen in private medical practice, but will also enable every physician to reach his or her highest possible level of professional competence and success.

Advantage and benefit of formal business education:

1. Physicians will have the tools to grow their medical practice business persistently and earn an unlimited amount of income that will give them the opportunity to enhance their medical skills and knowledge well beyond the average level we see today.

2. The extreme frustration permeating the medical profession today caused by the lack of appropriate and adequate professional income will be eliminated.

3. The increasing attrition of doctors caused by lack of the ability to earn the income necessary to meet their expectations will stop.

Conceptual argumentative points for providing a business education of all medical students are...

1. There is no lack of money in the world to do this.

2. There is no such thing as an impossible educational task that exceeds the comprehension and creativity of education scholars for making it happen.

3. It's time for the implementation of a formal academic business course that has been neglected for over a century in medical education. It is a critical issue necessary today for the survival of private medical practice.

"If future physicians were introduced to economic reality, the medical profession might cease to be part of the cost problem and become part of the solution."

-John G. Freymann, MD
National Fund for Medical Education

"By passionately targeting a business education, any business owner pulls back the curtain on an avalanche of alpha professional opportunities that would never be recognized otherwise. It's comparable to putting a mediocre jockey on a hell-of-a horse."

"The clear path to the bull's-eye of ultimate medical practice success is lit by business diligence, willful persistence, and self-discipline of the person you see in the mirror."

CHAPTER 1

The Reveal

"The Core Cause of the Disintegration of Private Medical Practice... and the One Remaining and Ignored Means of Preventing Its Extinction"

The story behind the cause began decades ago with the lack of a fundamental educational constituent required for the ultimate success and peak productivity of every physician whoever practiced medicine in our nation and those who are struggling and losing today because of it.

ALL MEDICAL STUDENTS understand that the process of becoming a medical doctor and practicing medicine is difficult and frustrating at times. Although that's the common view about being a physician, the view quickly expands into a nest of other unexpected and practice-destroying issues as students become more involved in the science and art of becoming a good physician.

What all medical schools seem to avoid telling students is how to face the more arcane challenges they will soon be facing and need to be prepared for.

The one great advantage medical students have that enables them to adapt to the whole truth about what they will be facing is their intense passion and desire to become a physician whatever it takes. After the first few years in medical practice, that same passion fades away and has to be transferred to another medical career objective.

Extremely traumatic consequences occur in the lives of physicians early in private medical practice when they begin to recognize that they should have been provided a business education all along in addition to their medical education.

Even fifty-two years ago, when I went through the medical school gauntlet, nothing was ever mentioned about the importance of knowing how to manage a medical practice business, let alone that it was critical to the outcome and to my goals.

Unfortunately, the same issue continues today in about 170 medical schools in our nation. In 2014 the importance of a business education for attaining one's peak potential as a physician has escalated to an unbelievable level, yet it escapes attention.

Most medical school academics still haven't caught on to the crucial importance of a business education for medical students and physicians. If they knew, then why haven't they done something about it already?

The tragedy of this neglect is both personal and profession-wide. Regardless of the possible reasons for the total lack of any obvious efforts that may have been proposed by medical education pundits to create a resolution, the ultimate damage caused by the continuing lack of any effectual solutions is visible.

Anyone who looks deeply enough into the present "practice-killer" conflicts found in the private practice of medicine (financial failure, extreme frustration with medical practice, and hopelessness felt among physicians who have practice problems and have no idea how to fix them) will recognize how severe the problem is. But more abusive issues than that are involved.

Without even giving any consideration to the business education of medical students being provided or required, the simple "necessity" of having a business education is not even mentioned, discussed, proposed, suggested, or superficially promoted by medical school academics and educators from their authoritative and responsible position.

This factor is even more reprehensible because the mindset of educational academics that reside and practice in the comforts and benefits of the secure environment of institutional medicine find it easy to disregard the reality faced by physicians outside that environment.

Ask any medical student or recently graduated young doctor if they were ever encouraged to obtain a business education during their training and education process. Students may occasionally hear a sidewalk mention of the need for a business education from occasional academics interested enough during the mentoring process to bring up the issue on a one-on-one basis. That sixty-second conversation usually only happens perhaps once over four years in medical school.

Is that something that any medical school should be proud of?

Understandably, students interpret the absence of a focused and direct promotion of business education repeatedly during their education as something that is not necessary or important to their medical career.

Such a stand should at least be shown to some degree by every educator and mentor coming into contact with students--and who cares enough about the degree of success of those medical students choosing a private medical practice career?

Other factors remain camouflaged in the medical academic world and often conflict with the basic ultimate goals of, and influence on, the later careers of medical students.

The following questions arise from a curious mind about medical education are:

1. Are the goals of medical school education today to *push medical students into employed positions* either in the managed care industry or in medical institutional medicine because they know we are headed towards socialized medicine anyway?

   That implies neglect of any concern for private practice issues.

2. In view of the major cause of present-day private medical practice financial failure, is it reasonable to doubt the necessity of a business education for every physician practicing today and in the future?

   This implies that financial failure of medical practice is of no concern to medical school education academics who feel *no responsibility* for resolving the problem.

3. Those who set the curriculum standards for medical school education are older and more experienced physicians and educational experts. Why is it not acceptable to realize that this group of educators is compromised by their experiential arrogance, fixed mindset, completely brainwashed by their own medical experiences, outdated knowledge about effective leadership, and personal biases they will never reveal to anyone?

   The issue here is, "Are these minds too saturated with ancient sticky beliefs and adherent bias factors that disqualify them for such decision making?"

4. Is there a widespread attempt by medical school educators to *intentionally neglect the business education issue* altogether? Could it be that they are so obsessed with packing more and more useless medical education into the heads of students that it doesn't allow time or room for business education, which is a much more critical issue to any private practice doctor?

   Someone is responsible for "piling on" excessive medical courses in medical school that go far beyond common sense and their usefulness to the majority of physicians. Take time to check the medical school curriculums today and make up your own mind!

Clear-thinking individuals with a desire to make a better life for all physicians (and their patients) must recognize the profound importance of providing every medical student graduating from medical school the widely recognized business tools and education proven to offer maximal success in the business of medical practice.

The purpose of this book is to arouse awareness within the medical education profession of the absolute necessity for every medical student to have a formal business education.

All physicians can make some money in private medical practice without much effort. But that accomplishment is short-lived in today's world of healthcare unless supported by a business education.

The lack of a formal business education is obviously the primary cause of financial failure of private medical practices. About every physician who agrees to sell his medical practice to the local hospital and becomes an employee of that hospital did it because of the urgent lack of enough medical practice income to keep his or her medical practice afloat.

In May 2014, the ability of any graduating medical student to reach an income level commensurate with attainment of their career goals and maintenance of their personal fulfillment can only be reached in private medical practice by using the tools provided by a formal business education.

No matter how smart or talented a doctor is in medicine, without a formal business education he or she will **never** reach his or her full career potential.

The business tools include marketing, effective management of practice and business, and business strategies known throughout the commercial business world as mandatory for any acceptable degree of success.

This is how the battle for the control of the healthcare system began and has continued to expand since.

Prior to 1960, fee for service in the practice of medicine had become the healthcare environment that made the medical profession desirable and attractive as a career.

Most medical students understood that a physician had the freedom to treat medical patients in their own manner unhindered by forces outside of medicine. This exploded their desire to go as far up the success ladder as they desired during their careers.

This upward momentum was not only possible but affordable for most. It was supported by a rapid escalation of medical technology. Better medical care was the result and no one complained. During the 1960s-1970s the costs of medical care increased dramatically because of the technological advances, but were accepted in light of better medical care. Older doctors remember this era of public criticism all too well.

Doctors became the scapegoats for the rising costs of healthcare. By the early 1970s managed care systems were born with the blessing of the government and large labor unions, and have since escalated in power, dominance, and authority regarding healthcare cost reduction and implementation.

This short and sketchy history reminds us of what has happened and changed in medical practice and healthcare over the last seven decades.

The real turning point for physicians began about 1970. At that time physicians in private practice were losing their patients in droves to the various managed care healthcare facilities.

Industry and unions that provided medical coverage for their employees and their families contracted with managed care facilities who guaranteed them that they would significantly reduce the cost of healthcare.

This began the gradual decline in medical practice revenue. Without agreeing to a 30 percent reduction in their usual medical fees, every doctor lost large numbers of their patients to managed care facilities. The later increase of guidelines, practice fee restrictions, and control of healthcare in many ways added another millstone to reliable medical practice income.

By the 1990s, the significant reduction in medical doctor incomes has become permanent and has been declining since. It means that physicians in general had been placed in a position where they could not do much of anything to increase their incomes other than working harder and seeing more patients (at least those without a business education).

There are two primary causes why physicians today are being forced out of private medical practice and hundreds are forced out of their medical careers:

1. Physicians have *never been taught how to efficiently and profitably manage the business of medical practice...* and never provided with a formal education in business and marketing.

2. Physicians have never been taught how and why to use the business and marketing tools proven *to keep them out of financial quicksand in the first place.*

Bottom line:

Physicians without a business education are predestined to fail financially in private medical practice, at least to some significant degree. Is that what every physician signed up for… a predictable financial failure of their medical practices?

An Odyssey of Generational Academic Indifference towards the Business Side of Private Medical Practice is Very Difficult to Rationalize or accept.

From 1800s to today *medical school curriculums have not been changed* to offer or to provide a business education for medical students. Any reasonably intelligent person can readily observe the evidence of private medical practice physician attrition resulting from lack of a business education.

If this isn't clear to you, then why are hundreds of medical doctors in our nation so willing to sell their personal medical practices to hospitals or close their practices and take on an indentured position of employment?

What realistic belief (and what situational factors are there that initiate that belief) are present that would cause any physician to give up their self-created independent medical practice business?

What powerful force would cause any doctor to give up their singular complete source of income that provides for their family and lifestyle for the rest of their lives in exchange for a practice lifestyle of employment where rules and restrictions of practice are made by the employer?

The psychological implications of being forced to give up personal control of their medical careers is a wound that destroys ambition, passion, and personal goals.

There are two obvious answers to these important questions: they can't earn enough money to meet their financial obligations and have no idea how to earn enough money to do it. It's all because they lack an academic business education.

What the general public (even physicians) doesn't know are the reasons why this is happening. That's because medical tradition prevents medical academics from exposing the issues involved regarding the need for a business education, which would otherwise make the medical educators appear negligent in their accountability.

Medical authorities who do know the causes and are in a position to resolve the problems associated with attrition of medical doctors do almost nothing to help resolve this catastrophic process.

They do know the importance of a business education for doctors, but forever procrastinate doing anything to help resolve this serious threat.

Surprisingly, the fact is that a large percentage of practicing doctors still don't recognize that the lack of a good business education leaves them *much more vulnerable to financial disaster*.

Even more surprising is the fact that less than one percent of physicians after medical school graduation will ever make a serious effort to obtain a business education, even after recognizing the need for it. Are physicians' simply reluctant martyrs and bushwhacked healers?

The easily visible and highly destructive factors and circumstances over the last five decades of medical practice in this nation should be enough to warrant actions within the healthcare system or medical education system to resolve it.

After seeing six decades of the slow degeneration of private medical practice, no one appears to actively be involved in eliminating the causes. There are several primary rationalizations for this aberrant behavior that seem to fit.

Probable reasons for such inaction and neglect are:

1. **Medical educators are stuck in the quicksand of tradition and doctrine.**

"It's the way it always been done and will continue to be done regardless of evidence to the contrary" is the attitude we see. If this is not the view of most medical educators with the power and position to do something, why hasn't the issue of providing a business education to medical students ever been initiated?

If such action would disturb the status-quo inertia of the present system, then it's not worth the benefits it offers in the first place... some feel. One of the most ironic implications of "tradition" is found in the definition of the word.

Tradition or dogma in a sense means, "A subtle unwritten means of telling you what you should accept and believe regardless of overwhelming evidence you shouldn't." Certainly, that definition is the exact opposite of what a professional medical education institution should stand for: an open mind and adaptation to constant change.

2. **Financial funding is lacking.**

There is no lack of money available in the world today. On March 7, 2014 the *Wall Street Journal* published an article and charts about wealth in this world today. Essentially, wealth is going up, not down. The problem is to find out where the money is and how to get it, not that it's hidden away somewhere and unreachable.

Isn't it interesting that almost all medical schools are endowed with large amounts of money and yet have no excess money to use to provide even the most superficial business education curriculum (estimated to be less than $500,000 to create and $200,000 to maintain each year).

For example, educational DVDs about business are the cheapest investments that can be made by medical schools for use by students. They can learn in their "off" times as a voluntary choice to learn business. However, digital media alone is certainly not the best choice.

Beginning a foundational business course (including marketing) within the medical school curriculum would not only increase the eventual financial productivity and skills of every medical school graduate but also add extraordinary recruiting value to the reputation of the school.

When business-educated physicians are able to earn far more revenue in private practice compared with today's physicians, they would also be in a predictable financial mode for donating much more money back to their alma mater.

Unfortunately, there seems to be a feeling among the elite medical schools in the nation that they graduate the most capable students who later become recognized and prestigious medical leaders and medical practice anointed physicians in the nation.

However, these medical schools never seem to recognize the far superior accomplishments that their graduates would make if they were also provided with an academic business education.

3. **Medical education curriculum is already overcrowded and medical students can't handle any more added education.**

It should be a "substitution" education process, not an "additional" education process.

No doubt some scholars believe that the medical student curriculum is already overcrowded with medical education requirements, and there's no room for teaching *non-medical courses.*

A close study of the medical education curriculums will reveal optional medical practice related areas of knowledge for medical students to learn that are unnecessary or superfluous to the usual private practice of medicine. Then it becomes a quandary as to which aspect of medical education is of more value to physicians over time.

Will a business education ever be a more valuable substitute for that other curriculum time that most physicians will never use? Yes, most private practice physicians know so. It doesn't require a survey of all private practicing physicians to document that.

Continuing to increase the amount of medical information that medical students are expected to learn during their medical education will become a significant beginning of the *educational burn-out process* that most will feel later during their careers… unless changes are made.

That single factor should be an over-the-top reason to selectively begin replacing the *medical "fringe" courses* mentioned above with the inherently more important and practical business education. It's something that is especially valuable to those medical students intending to enter private medical practice. It's also valuable to those who discover that practicing in an employment position is unsatisfactory and quit to start a private practice.

Medical schools and medical educators presently have a mindset for educating medical students to become so mentally fixated on employed positions, medical research, non-clinical careers, and "unit" or "group-oriented" medical decision making, that the impetus for accepting socialized medicine (a similar structure) has become an acceptable predisposition for every medical student.

This obvious step towards accepting socialized medicine is another step away from support for private medical practice by medical schools. Assuming that medical schools are planning ahead to be ready to adopt socialized medicine, the "business education" of medical students would be a useless effort.

The closer one gets to socialized medicine, the more respectable and advantageous it becomes emotionally, but not realistically.

Private medical practice is and always has been understood as being a small business entity. For any physician to be the most efficient and productive in private medical practice, they must have a business education. That's not debatable.

4. **A business education for medical students is totally unnecessary.**

The fact that the importance of business education is rarely if at all mentioned to medical students is ample evidence that medical school academics are…

a. Unwilling to establish or provide a business education even if they think it is needed in the private practice of medicine.

b. Denying that business knowledge has any advantage or value to private practice doctors.

c. Content with their present accomplishments in educating students only in medicine facts, information, and skills even though there are hundreds of financially failing medical practices increasing in numbers almost daily, which would not occur if all medical doctors had a formal business education.

d. Unaware or ignorant of what a business education truly provides for doctors in private medical practice. This question arises: Are medical education decision makers business ignorant and business uneducated? Or are they simply arrogant and unconcerned?

e. Admitting that physicians who are financially failing in private medical practice and those physicians who are unable to earn enough income to meet their full expectations from their careers is not the fault of medical school education scholars and is the fault of medical doctors themselves.

f. Admitting that they have no responsibility whatever to provide a business education for medical students even historically knowing that doctors will not obtain a business education on their own later.

g. Admitting that they are completely satisfied with the mediocre medical practice success and feeble accomplishments (described by the recognized business expert, Michael Gerber, who details those factors in his book, *The E-myth: Physician*) that the physicians they graduate from their medical school will have without the advantages that a business education provides.

h. Completely incompetent of ever being able to create an educational system that includes providing a business education of all medical students.

i. Certain that even though private medical practice is a real business and that business knowledge is a universal requirement for success, profitability, efficiency, productivity, growth, and management of medical practice… it does not require or suggest that medical school education scholars should have any responsibility to provide a business education.

j. Convinced that providing a formal business education for medical students during their four year medical education won't work, is impossible to do, or no one can come up with such a system.

It would be absurd to think that any of the above listed factors would hold any credibility in the academic world. However, the century-long disregard of the importance of a business education of doctors does bring up a serious concern about the diligence, if not the integrity, of all medical school academics.

If these things listed above have some level of truth to them, then the medical profession is disintegrating right under our eyes, because nothing will ever be done about resolving this issue.

This perpetuated myth that continues to be reinforced in the medical school communities has been fed so often to the medical students, overtly or covertly, that it has become the standard belief throughout the medical profession. This endless fiction has become the millstone around every physician's neck today. Even the intellectual exorcism of the myth by modern-day scholars has failed to rid us of the myth.

Barbara E. Kahn, professor of Marketing at the Wharton School of Business explains the search and thought sequencing of students, which I have adapted here to the need for a business education of medical students.

> *"The amount of search a student does is a function of an intuitive cost-benefit analysis. If a perceived benefit exists for taking the time and trouble to search for information, they will. If not, they stop at "good enough."*
>
> *When preconceived expectations do not exist, students will generally search more extensively before making a decision. New collected information is interpreted alongside existing information.*
>
> *Students take the information they already* think they know, *and tend to* reject information that runs counter to preconceived ideas, *called "confirmation bias."*

The point being made is that if medical school academics don't take time to *pre-educate* medical students about the cost-benefit aspects attributed to a business education of physicians, then students will never take the advice seriously.

If they don't implant the benefits of a business education in their minds and don't provide students with reasonable preconceived expectations of a business education (as an introduction to actually getting a business education that a medical school should provide for them), students will often reject the idea of a business education being necessary.

5. **Medical students will not tolerate any business education plan.**

Business education must be a *fixed educational process* within the medical school curriculum. It's not a voluntary choice for students.

Medical school academic curriculums for medical students are "fixed" for them, especially in the first two years of medical school. Therefore, students never realize what they might have been missing out on at the time. In any education system, students should be told at the beginning what they should learn from the education system.

It means that they should be told about the importance and advantages of having a business education. Are they told? *No.*

Most intelligent educators know what happens when students are never informed about everything (especially about business) they need to learn. Students in this scenario (not knowing anything about what a business education can do for them in medical practice) end up with having only one focus: to learn medical knowledge and skills.

That intense distraction of their focus only on medical learning has the same effect on student's minds as an experienced pilot has when landing with his "wheels-up." The loud gear horn blasting in his ears, telling him that he is about to crash land, is completely consciously ignored by the brain, in spite of the danger.

The fact that the brain fed by all the senses takes in, stores away, and accumulates an estimated two billion bits of information about the world every day tends to invalidate the argument about students not being able to handle the extra learning load.

No proof exists that there is a limitation to the amount of learning the brain can handle. A photographic mind that few people are gifted with supports the "no-limitations factor" of the brain's capacity.

Alternatives to lightening the educational load.

Another present increasing trend in the medical profession today of splitting-off or subdividing specialties of medical practice into more manageable education and training capabilities has, maybe even without intent, established a means to manage and reduce the overwhelming amount of increasing medical information that students and doctors are required to learn and apply.

Here is a pertinent example, about dividing the OB-GYN specialty into separate OB and GYN components, which I expect to happen soon, for several reasons.

The rising malpractice risks associated with obstetrical practice today has destroyed many OBG specialists. Any number of malpractice suits filed against physicians, whether valid or settled outside the court, often result in denial of state licensures, denial of malpractice insurance coverage, and financial loss of medical practices (tough to earn enough in GYN practice alone after stopping OB practice).

Dividing the two specialties would enable those doctors in Gyn to avoid the much higher risks associated with obstetrical practice as well as avoid the associated assumption of medical gyn incompetency made about doctors who practice both Ob and Gyn whenever an obstetrical malpractice case comes around. If a doctor is incompetent in obstetrics, he or she probably is also incompetent in gynecology practice, is the thought.

Allowing medical students to choose which medical and clinical curriculum courses to take (like they did in college) would result in medical education chaos. Medical education scholars lock medical students into a fixed regimen of education because academic scholars know the most efficient and productive medical learning sequence for their professional education.

Students don't know what they need to learn in medical school, so they *have to be told*. Medical academics, understandably, don't want their curriculums messed with by adding business education to the medical curriculum even if they aren't the business instructors who teach it.

This insinuates that *medical practice business is less important than clinical medical practice*. For the permanently *employed* physician, it's true.

For students headed for private medical practice, it's wrong thinking. For the survival of private medical practice, business education is critically important for physicians, especially in the present economic environment and political intrusions into medicine.

Another way to look at this business education process.

Medical students have been led to believe that being a physician deserves a "promised land" of their own. It hasn't happened yet.

To get there, the older generations of medical academics have now disappeared. Therefore, it's the perfect time to create and implement an *academic business education course* into the medical school curriculum.

Because I have not lived or practiced close enough to the medical educational academic environment over the past forty-five or so years,

I recognize my shortfall of medical education knowledge and the many reasons medical education today continues on with its own educational shortfall.

The response I would expect from the medical education academics would lie somewhere between, "If we could have included a business education for medical students and felt it was important enough, we would have done so" and "There are limits to what we are able to do within the medical school educational system which makes such a business education addition to the present curriculum impossible." Garbage thinking, I believe.

I refuse to accept the idea that the whole medical school education system is so rigidly fixed in concrete relative to business education of students that it can't be significantly improved. By teaching new doctors how to use business education tools to expand their incomes, it provides them with an unlimited ability to continually upgrade their skills, medical knowledge, and ultimate potential in medical practice.

And I haven't even mentioned the outstanding reputation and elite positioning it places the medical school in, especially ones that are the first to graduate young doctors with such a high caliber of medical practice potential.

Why wouldn't every medical school see the fantastic advantage of graduating such advanced and business educated medical professionals who would dramatically upgrade our national healthcare system… as well as significantly improve their own incomes and medical practice satisfaction, and make the present "professional poverty" a thing of the past?

I'm sure that the politicians (government) would love to usurp the benefits derived by their control of this explosive adventure into new medical education territory.

It's my firm belief that such a business education addition, regardless of the simplicity or complexity of the business education system created, would be a perfect starting point. It's something that gradually can be improved upon to match the capability level of every graduating medical student that any medical school intends to focus on.

This program would be less intrusive to implement than a hybrid MD + PhD program that some medical schools already have. However, a business education program would be especially beneficial to many more physicians in private medical practice... even more so, an important factor for saving private medical practice itself.

Most educational scholars understand that if a student is thirsty for knowledge, a student will grab whatever looks good and figure it out later. The perfect time when students are in that frame of mind is when they are in medical school. Consequently, most students would be in that frame of mind to accept the business education curriculum without having to be talked into it.

Any ambitious and motivated medical student, once knowledgeable about what a business education empowers them to do in their medical career, should be smart and mature enough to visualize their future in medicine as more productive, more controllable, and more adaptable to their personal career expectations.

How valuable is this? That depends on the student.

Its value to medical schools can only come from your use of what I show you and let you in on in this treatise and followed by the implementation of a formal business education process.

Those who disregard this business education process, in my opinion, suffer from gross intellectual laziness and have not given this even half a chance to prove its value. We are talking here about the *complete education* of medical students (both medical and business) in a laudable effort to graduate medical doctors who are fully capable of meeting every challenge they will face in private medical practice in the future... **which virtually all doctors today lack.**

"Our future is preordained by our past unless we intervene in the present."
-Dan S. Kennedy

"Motivation is the art of getting people to do what you want them to do because they want to do it."
---Dwight Eisenhower

CHAPTER 2

The Problem

"The Educational Wound that Handicaps All Physicians Right from the Start"

Predestined financial business failure of physicians in the private practice of medicine epitomizes the extent to which medical school education academics are willing to go to escape responsibility to provide a formal business education of all medical students, thus *seriously compromising* the *maximum potential* of every private practicing physician in this nation today.

AS OF OCTOBER 2014, to my knowledge not a single one of the reported 170 or so medical schools in our nation provides or offers formal business education to their medical students. Furthermore, there is unfortunately little effort to do so much as to encourage or even advise medical students about the necessity and importance of a business education to their medical career.

Consequently, every private practicing physician today is left to "try" to efficiently and hopefully also profitably run their medical practice business with little or no knowledge about such things as business management, marketing, and the many requirements necessary for success of any business. If ever there was a seemingly essential profession doomed to suffer financially, this is it.

The evidence of this unacceptable situation is extensive and substantiated by increasing physician attrition and extreme frustration with their medical careers.

One may excuse this oversight by medical educators of the essential need for the business education of physicians, but not the intentional avoidance of providing a formal business education of medical students.

This is especially true when the supposed educational goal is to create medically smart physicians with a fully engaged capacity to build and expand their professional career (professional business) while using the foundation of medical practice business to accomplish that end.

The fact is that the private practice of medicine is a business-validated legally established business entity.

When medical education academics then declare themselves as not being responsible for anything more than a medical education of medical students, it's a daring and aggressive stance that trends outside of their moral compass and due diligence.

So here we are today expected to get into line to congratulate the seminal architects of the medical school education dynasty for a job well done when hidden behind this medical education façade is an educational shortcoming that boggles the minds of highly regarded business experts around the world.

Nothing is as devastating to the minds and souls of physicians as one day recognizing that they have been sent out into the world to accomplish miracles in medical practice and discover that they are devoid of a business education required to accomplish those miracles.

Does anyone believe that physicians can run a profitable medical practice while learning business principles and strategies along the way (as most physicians do today)? Of course they can and do somehow by the grace of God. But there's a relentless bullet hole in this seemingly self-sufficient belief that has been fostered by the medical schools for over a century. Medical school academics "know" and believe that it doesn't require a business education.

Most everyone knows that the great majority of all doctors make good money in medical practice because they drive new cars, have nice homes, and raise families on their practice income.

It's what the business expert and author Michael Gerber calls "mediocre medical practices" that nearly all medical doctors eventually settle for. Not what they want, but what they are willing to accept because they are ignorant of their alternatives that can rapidly improve their circumstances.

This surrender to professional mediocrity is the destructive essence that's destroying private medical practice today.

What the general public and most all patients don't know is that in exchange for their $200,000 investment (and debt) in education, a significant number of doctors work in a job that earns much less than many high school graduates, who move up in job ranks over time.

The public does not know or understand that doctors' incomes have been steadily dropping over the last thirty years and will continue to drop as a result of government fee restrictions.

The most devastating factor relating to doctor's incomes is that they are led to believe they don't need a business education. That's because they don't know what they don't know and rely on their "superb genius" to solve their financial problems for themselves.

What doctors don't know is what advantages a formal business education adds to their medical career success. They have to be told. There is no debate that virtually all physicians with a business education are capable of tripling their private medical practice income using that knowledge. The other more important advantages are discussed in chapter 5.

Up to this point, I have been discussing issues that pertain only to private medical practice physicians. A view about what happens to employed physicians under these circumstances is also relevant.

Employed physicians who become unemployed and then go into private medical practice (about 15 percent of employed doctors) are faced with the same need for business education.

With the trend of salaries and practice incomes of medical doctors on a downward swing over the last three decades or more, hospitals cutting medical staff positions to cut costs, the overall national economy at bankruptcy level, and the expected disappearance of private medical practice because of our government-controlled healthcare, one would expect to see even more serious medical career problems for most all physicians in the future.

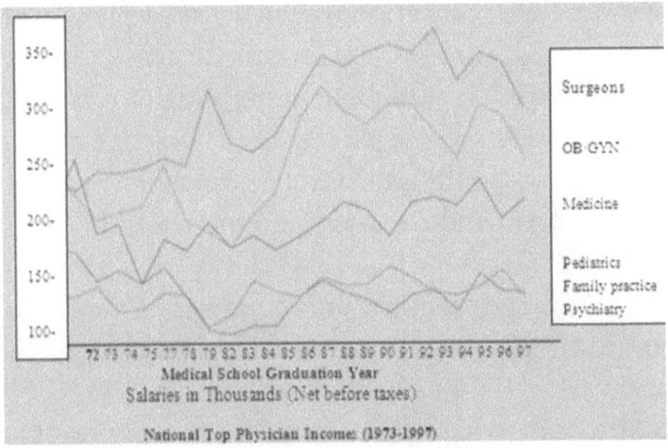

This then begs the following questions:

1. Who then is responsible for the additional business education of medical students… medical schools or students themselves?

2. Who or what entity will stand up and make this necessary business education a reality regardless of the circumstances and barriers that need to be overcome in doing so?

3. The incredibly weak responses physicians have made over the last fifty years to prepare themselves with even a reasonable business education after medical school graduation show that physicians just won't do it on their own.

   Other than on-the-job training (like most doctors use to start their practices), one should ask whether there is any important reason a doctor even needs a business education. Or is it "good enough" to let doctors remain ignorant of the management benefits of knowing how to run a medical practice business profitably for the duration of their careers?

4. How is it possible to include a business education course into the curriculum of medical schools when medical students are already deluged with an avalanche of often-never-used medical knowledge? Could there be a few efficient ways to do it without compromising a medical student's time and school requirements for learning medicine?

5. Has the medical education system given up pursuing the effort to educate physicians destined for private medical practice and has now complied with the political agenda to educate all medical doctors to become employees... where the doctor's medical knowledge and skills are severely restricted while working under the direction of and responsibilities to the ubiquitous employer?

Of course, these questions are only a few of the many that are under consideration in this report and are discussed further in chapter 4.

Evidence that should ignite a nationwide earth-shaking mandate for educating medical students in more things than the accumulation of medical knowledge.

The fact that almost all physicians never realize that they are severely "business" compromised throughout their medical careers today means that the business side of medical practice is completely ignored by medical academics.

The earth-shaking thought that medical students (and later as physicians) never recognize that they have far more capabilities and potential than they ever imagined for learning business along with medicine is so eloquently described in the book, *The E-myth: Physician,* written by the renowned business expert Michael Gerber.

As a result of consulting with his many doctor clients it became obvious to Mr. Gerber that all physicians function in a giant nebula of assumed competence in running their business of medical practice, while in fact they are wallowing around in, at best, a mediocre and inefficient business. Evidence of that speaks for itself.

In today's medical practice environment, where financial failures of hundreds of private medical practices are happening monthly and physicians are seeking employment, one has to ask why this is happening. There are two openly credible causes that nearly all business experts would agree with.

1. The present-day "relative poverty stricken" physicians are situated in is due not only because of practice and medical fee restrictions to begin with, but also because physicians who realize that they are in financial trouble with their practices have

no business tools to use that could very well have prevented the issue or reversed their financial situation if they had had a formal business education.

2. The perpetual medical school enigma and stance against the provision of a business education of students is causing indisputable harm to every medical school graduate.

   Even the fact that medical schools are making no significant effort to stress to the students the necessity of business knowledge and the importance of it, implies that they mistakenly believe students are smart enough to already know it--and really aren't.

   Second, and the more important consequence, is that without being fully informed about the above factors about business, medical students will inevitably interpret the subliminal message from their medical school that business knowledge doesn't offer a significant advantage to doctors.

   Therefore, students have no motivation or desire to seek a business education sometime later in their career. And it never reaches the level of desire necessary to do it. The inspirational seed is never planted during medical school.

A foundational truth:

Every successful business owner knows and understands the necessary requirements for success in any business. Why don't doctors?

Business principles all physicians should know, remember and use in their private medical practice.

1. **The same business principles are applicable to every kind, size, and purpose that exists for a business entity. The late business education pioneer Peter Drucker described a business purpose as "to get customers and keep them."**

   The business knowledge-handicapped person is impressed with the erroneous thought that his business is "different" and doesn't respond to the accepted standard business principles… Baloney!

Certainly the scope and application of each business principle varies with the objective and circumstances, thereby requiring a continuous adaptation of the business process in stepwise fashion to remain successful.

2. **The use of business systems accounts for the highest level of income, productivity, efficiency, and ultimate business success.**

Superior business systems are composed of a series of sequential processes required to accomplish each segment of the final product. Those processes are highly organized and detailed so that any new worker can walk into that job process and know exactly how to do it because the process is the same regardless of previous work experience.

The best example of that is like the characteristics of an industrial "assembly line." The same systems can be created by a physician for every job duty in the medical office, which eliminates conflicts of job responsibilities, wasting of time, and the commonly found bickering among employees.

The world's most sought after business and marketing expert, Dan S. Kennedy, teaches: that *"Ultimately, successful businesses can't be run by committee or consensus."*

3. **Business efficiency requires knowledgeable business management and employees who are educated in the importance of their job duties, supervised, compatible with team efforts, and are informed of the employer's ultimate goals.**

The greatest mistake made in business today, especially in medical practice offices, is depending on employees to work towards the employer's primary objectives, automatically have a work ethic focused on the employer's expectations, and understand their obligations in the team effort without ever being told or informed why.

Exposing your inner thoughts to a bunch of your uninterested employees is difficult. Erma Bombeck says, "It takes a lot of courage to show someone else your dreams."

Even the well-known business author Robert Kiyosaki calls business a "team sport."

4. **The highest productivity of any business depends on the efficiency and reliability of the business systems that are in place.**
   Efficiency is the ideal factor for increasing productivity. In business, both are required elements of a high success level.

"The willingness to do whatever it takes is infinitely more important than knowing everything there is to know about how to do it."
-Dan S. Kennedy

5. **The optimal success of any business depends on how effectively business principles are used to expand the business.**
   The essential issue for physicians is to know and learn how to use these principles in ways that are practical, efficient, and profitable.

"No matter how great your ability, how large your genius, or how extensive your education, your achievement will never rise higher than the confidence you have in yourself."
-Lee Milteer, author and speaker

6. **The ultimate outcome of any business effort depends entirely on the capacity of that business to take all actions necessary to accumulate interested customers, persuade them to buy in to the services, products, or activities, and continuously maintain that business relationship as long as possible.**
   For the business of medical practice this translates to a significant and perpetual effort by physicians to attract new patients in the amount necessary to provide adequate revenue to meet all objectives.
   Adequate revenue for the business implies an income level that pays all business expenses and an additional income level that appropriately provides for the continuing education and

improvement of training and skills to maintain the level of competency that keeps a physician at the top of his profession.

Adequate revenue means that the profits made are proportional to the level of want or need that the physician requires to maintain a chosen lifestyle, personal and family objectives.

"I don't believe you have to be better than everybody else. I believe you have to be better than you ever thought you could be."
---Ken Venturi

7. **Strategic and targeted continuous marketing and advertising as well as the appropriate use of every promotional tactic for the business are the primary drivers for the success of any business.**

It's what every doctor must do to ensure that his or her medical practice is continuously growing, income is increasing without interruption, and the financial support of a physician's career and goals, both personal and medical practice-wise, are secured.

Without business and marketing knowledge, every physician is predisposed to the destructive potential of every threat known to compromise any business entity in existence. Because almost all physicians are never taught foundational business principles, they are sitting ducks for failure at some level of medical practice.

"To achieve much of anything....
that must be your mindset....
Remember, it's all my own choice."
-Dan S. Kennedy

8. **All businesses must be sensitive to and adapt to continuous changes in economic cycles, demands of customers, trends in buying habits of customers, competition pressures, and governmental control of healthcare, among others.**

The business of medical practice is no different. In our medical world, patients have moved from being willing to believe and accept a doctor's advice and treatment to the present generation of patients who are in control of their own healthcare.

Physicians today face the conflict between ethical and submissive forms of advice and treatment as a result of the power of patient demands. Unhappy patients move elsewhere, spread bad stories, and start lawsuits.

This adaptation process is not something that is taught in medical school. It's a learn-as-you-go process.

However, a business education provides strategies, ideas, and training that enable doctors to adapt to the changes more quickly, efficiently, and productively, leaving them in full control of their medical business. Therefore, physicians are in a position to remain in authority while providing agreeable alternatives.

9. **A fundamental principle behind the success of any business is that there are established and reliable measurements of every parameter of the business process made that confirm the direction, growth or decline of the productivity of the business.**

Almost all physicians over the past century and even today have no realistic idea about how to measure the important elements of their medical practice business, what those elements are, and what the measurements tell them.

In essence, most all medical doctors at any point in time have no documentation of how their medical practice is doing. Most doctors take a casual look at their monthly financial statement and at the net income figure without any thought that that income figure is a result of the intermittent receivables scattered over several months and of billing efforts that just happened to show up as income this month.

Ask any doctor to give you a thorough review of what his monthly financial statement is showing them and he can't. Even the simplest method of measuring how the medical practice is doing—that of keeping a record of every new patient coming in and every old patient leaving their practice—is a rarity.

A business education is meant to ease all that pain. Business expert Peter Drucker says, "What gets measured, gets done."

10. **Another business principle embedded in the minds of successful business owners is the need for a business mindset. That mindset, attitude, focus, and passion for business success has to be equal to the passion they have for dominance in their professional career.**

    Unfortunately, for most physicians their passion for their medical career has already taken hold of their brain so strongly that the importance of having business knowledge is at the bottom of the bucket.

    That's a prominent reason a formal business education of medical students should be taught at that level of integrated thinking when the brain can handle both medical and business learning. It's the same mental adaptation that one experiences in learning a second or third language.

"Plans are only good intentions unless they degenerate into hard work."
-Peter Drucker

Many specific benefits that business-knowledgeable physicians have over physicians that don't are:

1. The ability to create a highly efficient and productive medical practice office.

2. Business-wise doctors are much more aware of oncoming trends, economic surges, and external business forces that directly affect their medical business. Seeing those things earlier than others enables them to stay ahead of the herd with all the early advantages associated with it.

3. Business-wise doctors make significantly more income during their medical careers than others. The difference has been estimated to be about $1 million.

4. Business-wise doctors are more knowledgeable and skillful because they can afford the extra training and education all doctors seek.

5. Business-wise doctors are more in demand by patients because of their superior skills and knowledge. They can afford to obtain those attributes.

6. Business-wise doctors maintain an elevated status in the professional community.

7. Business-wise doctors are the preferred doctors that other doctors refer their patients to more often.

8. Business-wise doctors have more advantages for promoting their medical practices and so have larger practices and income.

9. Business-wise doctors have more money to spend on marketing their practices, so they earn more income.

10. Business-wise doctors are usually the happiest and least frustrated about medical practice problems. Have you ever met a wealthy doctor who is always complaining? They are rare indeed.

The disadvantages that result from the *lack* of a formal business education of physicians are the following:

1. Physicians fail to see imminent business problems approaching soon enough to prepare for them or even prevent them.

2. Physicians don't know the lessons of marketing that would permit them to prevent the financial failure of their medical practice.

3. Physicians have no adequate knowledge about how marketing works, how to use marketing appropriately, and don't comprehend the value that it adds to their medical practice business.

4. Physicians have no adequate knowledge about business which over the last fifty years is primarily responsible for our present-day attrition of physicians.

5. Physicians are unable to track how their medical practice business is doing because they don't know how to measure the status of their business.

6. Physicians resort to working harder to make money instead of knowing how to work less and make more income using business tools.

7. Physicians fail to understand marketing strategies for improving their medical business.

8. Physicians are always behind in their practices and are always having to play catch-up to others who already have business knowledge and skills.

9. Once physicians finally recognize that their medical practice is financially failing, it's often too late to save it.

10. **The following are** problems with setting up a medical practice *without business knowledge*:

    a. Not considering demographics when picking a place to start medical practice.

    b. Long-term consequences related to future medical practice changes are not considered.

    c. Don't know how to recruit the best patients or how to market for new patients.

    d. Don't understand how to set attainable goals that are part of a career plan to reach the top.

e. Rarely have any written business plans to follow, and don't recognize at the time the value and advantages of having a written business plan.

f. Don't apply real *due diligence* to much of anything.

"There are certain desires and emotional triggers that motivate people to suspend logic and critical thought and that are so universal that the age, education, financial status, and etc. of the consumer doesn't matter."

---Dan S. Kennedy

CHAPTER 3

The Pain

"The Inevitable Educational Trauma that Keeps Driving Physicians Out-of Private Medical Practice"

Lack of an academic business education is the core cause of financial failure of doctors in private medical practice.

EVERY MEDICAL SCHOOL education scholar should develop true understanding of the torment and distress imposed on physicians by the lack of an academic business education during the medical school educational process.

The fact that the attrition rate of medical doctors today is at its highest in the history of medical practice, should concern everyone.

It's also the only time in history of the medical profession that the severe disappointment and frustration of over 50 percent of private practicing physicians (recent AMA survey) are seriously considering leaving active medical practice. Something must be done immediately to resolve the problem—everyone knows that—but no one is doing much about it, if anything.

So why isn't there a massive effort already in progress today aimed at correcting this obvious cause: the lack of a formal business education?

The painful financial wounds that private practice medical doctors are desperately trying to placate today have neither affordable nor vicarious solutions available to them.

Unfortunately, most private practicing physicians see only one primary solution to their distress with their medical careers… quitting medical practice.

Quitting medical practice is at the top of the list because physicians don't know, nor have ever been shown or told about any other reasonable or effective means for reducing the overwhelming stress and disappointment caused by their professional poverty. Most physicians do understand that they still have one remaining income increasing alternative… working harder and seeing more patients, a short-lived path to burnout.

Of course, working harder increases the practice stress to the point of burnout and triples the problems associated with trying to quickly attract many more new patients when they have no idea how to do that efficiently or effectively. More time with patients leads to less time at home and increasing family conflicts.

Piled on top of their persistent struggle with those issues is the fact that almost every physician subconsciously understands that these income-destroying factors could be resolved if they only had the business knowledge to make it happen. Physicians know, but remain in denial about the absolute necessity of knowing how to run their medical practice business much more successfully, to make more money and to resolve the primary cause of their dilemma: lack of adequate income.

All the stress factors above are related to making enough income to enable them to reach all of their professional goals and secure their family obligations. Do they stop practicing and go get the business education they need?

Rarely does any physician in private medical practice compromise their already insufficient medical practice income in order to pay the estimated $40,000 for an elite MBA education that may not by itself be enough to put the medical practice back in the black, financially. An MBA will not guarantee that result, but is a good start.

It's too much of a stretch to accept for almost all physicians. Medical school educators look at this practice destroying scenario and irresponsibly conclude that, *"It's their own responsibility to get the business education they need on their own time. And if they financially fail in their medical practice, it's their problem, not ours."*

Medical school educators, already knowing what will probably happen to most doctors who are practicing in financially unstable practices, continue to disregard their own obligations to "fully prepare" physicians they educate to manage a professional practice business profitably.

In reality, medical school educators, already knowing what will probably happen to most of these doctors (mediocre or worse medical practice financial stability) continue to disregard their own obligations to fully prepare the physicians they educate to manage a professional practice business profitably.

Medical schools and medical educators, the decision makers, have yet to accept that medical education is a changed reality. A hundred years ago medical education served physicians well enough. Today medical education requires an education that encompasses a business education for any private practice physician to make a reasonable or far higher income from practice, depending on their ambition and persistence.

But in the eyes of all the physicians who have been or are now suffering from the lack of a formal business education (specifically, financially failing medical practices), medical educators are ethically and morally truly responsible for providing that business education during medical school education regardless of the barriers associated with doing so.

Most disturbing is the position taken by over 170 medical schools. They have apparently decided that it's acceptable under any standards of educational judgment to graduate medical students who are incompletely prepared for private medical practice and for running a medical practice business. The complete neglect of the business side of medical practice by medical school educators is a dishonor to the profession and an enigma that can't be supported by any intellectually responsible community of educators.

"The physician is expected to meet the grim monster, break the jaws of death, and pluck the spoil out of his teeth."

-R. V. Pierce, MD, (1895)
President: World's Dispensary Medical Association, Buffalo, NY

The real causes of physician discontent are often not what you may think!

1. **Inadequate income compensation** (top of the list)

The overwhelming emotional toll on the lives of every practicing physician today due to inadequate income is the number one and most logical contributing cause for most of a doctor's frustration with medical practice.

Lack of money to pave the way to a doctor's professional fulfillment and satisfaction with their medical career begins and ends with their dependence on earnings that enable it all. Money enables us to do almost everything we ever want to do with our professional lives.

Lack of adequate income compromises goals previously set, creates the need for readjustments of one's medical career downwards, and requires downgrading one's lifestyle inside and outside the medical community. Those financial factors have a profound impact on every doctor's perspective about their medical career as well as a measurement of their success.

Another very emotional pulse-pounder that wears down self-esteem is the fact that physicians frequently aren't able to provide their family with all they had promised and that the family members expected.

Such things as a decent college education for the children, ability to fully fund a retirement program, and the ability to fulfill the expected and promised advantages both to themselves and their families are often out of reach.

The root cause of this scenario lies with the fact that a physician (without a business education) never becomes cognizant of the business tools available that not only prevents, but also can reverse bad financial situations before circumstances reach the point of no return.

There is a point of no return in every private medical practice, where all the forces and strategies of business knowledge cannot prevent complete financial failure of the medical practice.

For most physicians without a business tools library in mind, recognition of the downward collapse and ultimate financial failure comes too late to recover.

Now, we often see disturbing numbers of medical practice failures that increasingly substantiate the necessity for a formal business education for medical students. Physicians already in medical practice won't do it. And the most practical time for business education instruction is during the medical school education curriculum to ensure they get a business education.

Such an educational neglect is devastating to all concerned, especially when there is a business education cure right out there waiting to be recognized and implemented into all private medical practices today.

Undoubtedly, every medical doctor with a formal business education under their belt will find a time and place to use everything they learned to great advantage over all others who ignore it.

"Much disappointment, frustration, and failure can be traced to the fool's mission of finding a single, simple solution to a complex problem or opportunity." *-Dan S. Kennedy*

Lack of adequate professional practice income and not knowing how to significantly increase their income, often results in the separation of a physician from their family and family obligations. It, in turn, often results in major family crises including divorce, mental problems like depression or worse and even loss of passion for their medical career. Bankruptcy and a continuing presence in the mind of many conflicts that are associated with financial problems can often last for years to come.

The lack of adequate private practice income also directly affects a physician's attention to their medical practice. Interference with the ability to communicate well with patients, inability to manage the medical practice efficiently, and making medical mistakes are all common consequences of the lack of a formal business education.

In order to better understand the full benefit that an adequate income means to every private practice physician, consider the logical impact of this sequence to medical practice income:

a. A physician in private medical practice must earn enough profit from the practice to cover all personal and business expenses and to remain in the business of medical practice.

b. The source of all medical practice income is earned by seeing, treating, and advising enough medical patients to be profitable as a business.

c. When income is adequate, physicians can afford to obtain any and all medical education and training programs to continually advance their competence and skills. Doctors with poor incomes can't afford to obtain these advancements to maintain their medical competence.

d. When income is adequate, doctors are able to provide for all family needs and obligations.

e. When physicians are able (know how to) to propel their income and obtain superior education and training during their medical practice careers, they become much better doctors. They are more valuable to their medical patients, are much more in demand, will build a larger practice, and earn more income, and the cycle is perpetuated.

f. This earning cycle of growth and increasing income is not related to how hard a physician works or how many hours are spent in the hospital and office each day as is commonly thought. Long hours and hard work often results in burnout, a career destroying factor.

The revolving earning cycle that continuously floods the practice with new patients over the duration of each medical career of every private practice doctor is powered by the *continuous application and implementation of business strategies and tools, like marketing.*

"All businesses succeed or die on the effectiveness of their marketing systems."
-Dan S. Kennedy

2. Governmental restrictions on medical practice.

A brief background history of how we ended up in this present professional financial quicksand is pertinent.

Although the "progressive movement" idea of our national government about controlling healthcare dates as far back as Harry Truman, the **wake-up call for physicians hit home in the late 1960s and early 1970s.**

Finally, numerous complaints about the rapidly rising costs of healthcare by the large labor unions and industrial giants convinced Congress to approve the creation of "managed care" medical care organizations.

These new medical organizations promised to quickly reduce the rapidly rising healthcare costs by contracting with major business and labor union groups who were covering (paying for) the healthcare of their employees.

By doing that, managed care groups were given the power to become controllers of medical care offered to patients who belonged to these industry segments.

Once the managed care facilities were certified, they needed to find medical doctors to care for the patients. They contracted with local area doctors to provide medical care. It was necessary to convince medical doctors to signup to provide medical care for the managed care contracted patients. They cleverly did it with the use of two ingenious, yet arcane strategies.

First, by promising to supply the private doctors who signed up with a managed care group a constant flow of new patients. In essence, the thought was that a physician might double or triple the size of his present medical practice and income by making that move.

Second, by convincing those physicians who signed up to treat the managed care patients, the increased volume of patients they theoretically would get would more than compensate every doctor for agreeing to accept a significantly lower professional fee pay schedule (about 30 percent lower) that the managed care groups offered.

For physicians hoping to build their private practice faster, make their medical practice more competitive in the local community, and increase their practice income even above the usual level of income earned by doctors in their area, the opportunity certainly seemed very desirable over the long haul.

What sounded good for physicians in the beginning quickly turned sour later, so what happened?

A. *Contracted physicians* discovered that a constant and perpetual battle with the managed care facilities was necessary to order, prescribe, treat and do things that beforehand they had had the freedom to do… and now couldn't.

Doctors had to order medication for patients that were on the managed care formulary. Drugs that were not on the managed care formulary, patients had to pay for out-of-pocket. If the contracted physician did not prescribe formulary drugs for patients, the patients, refusing to pay for medication themselves, often moved to a contracted doctor who would.

Doctors were limited in their selection of surgical procedures and lab testing as well. All had to be approved by managed care personnel first, meaning that they controlled the procedures done on their patients and the lab tests ordered, further reducing the freedom that those private (contracted) doctors had to practice under.

B. *Non-contracted physicians* found the lowering of medical fees and having them dictated to them from the managed care groups was totally unacceptable and refused to see and treat the managed care patients. They discovered quickly that their loyal patients were dropping out of their practices in significant numbers to move to a contracted doctor, as required by their managed care healthcare system.

If they didn't do it, they would be forced to pay for all healthcare services out-of-pocket to their non-contracted doctors.

For many physicians in private practice who lost patients because their patients were required to move to a contracted doctor, it not only financially crippled many of those medical practices, but also resulted in financial failure of many of those practices.

Every medical doctor with a business education is able to quickly and much earlier recognize the devastating effects that the predictable loss of so many patients would create for their own practices and upgrade their marketing for recruiting more patients.

These business knowledgeable doctors would have started a massive new patient recruiting process (called "marketing" their practices) early enough to prevent the possible coming disaster.

However, physicians in the 1970s *had no business education* background and were left to suffer the full consequences of the loss of up to half of their original patient load. I was practicing then and it wasn't pretty. At first I resisted joining these managed care groups because of their practice restrictions. It wasn't long before I changed my mind and joined them all, but it didn't really increase my income.

Contracted physicians were not permitted to refer their patients to non-contracted physicians either for consultation or treatment, with few exceptions.

In a geographical area where a non-contracted physician consultant practiced and where there was no other similar contracted physician consultant available within one hundred miles of the referring physician, the local consultant was usually approved and paid for the patients care provided.

Physicians lost the one major source of new medical patients: referrals from other doctors. *Research has documented that over 60 percent of new patients arriving at a medical practice originate from other doctor's referrals.*

It eventually became a *survival necessity* for a majority of physicians to sign-up with regional managed care entities whether they liked it or not.

The sucking away of so many medical patients by managed care groups almost destroyed the existence of private medical practice. Today the same situation exists, but for different reasons.

Today, new and older medical doctors are being forced into becoming employees on salary because they, like before, can't make enough income to stay in private medical practice.

C. **The triumph of complexity over common sense status for physicians.**

The repugnant coercion strategy of the U.S. government to force physicians to comply with the government mandate of managed care became the first strategic step in the progressive agenda for full control of health care.

Eventually, most physicians became servants of the restrictive governmental managed healthcare mandate. Only a small segment of other physicians managed to continue practicing independent of the mandate, but those who did were by necessity forced to go to extremes to maintain and grow their practices (without a business education to guide them).

For most physicians in these circumstances, complying fully with the managed care system led to unacceptable consequences, such as:

1. The mandate was extended to include Medicaid and Medicare patients, further decreasing the available medical patient population for doctors that remained outside the managed care system.

2. Both the contracted and non-contracted physicians discovered that their practice incomes were slowly decreasing at about 1 percent overall per year, and has continued to this day. (AMA survey, physician's salaries—1973-1997: see graph on page 36.)

3. A *physician's lack of a formal business education* that would have given all doctors an opportunity over all those years to recover financially can be addressed by using all of the time-proven successful business strategies and tools.

   The result of the effort would today be far superior to their actual deplorable circumstances all physicians continue to embrace today. Living in relative "professional poverty" is definitely not what any doctor expects from their medical career choice.

Would you think that physicians today are smart enough to recognize that jumping off of the speeding medical practice train about to crash would be a smart move? Maybe!

After all the time involved, money spent, and intense efforts to become a physician (and now, on top of all the other obligations including extreme educational debts piled on), this qualifies as an insurmountable deterrent to the choice of a medical career today.

So every doctor is thinking today, "Is it worth the effort? Can I tolerate working that hard with those medical practice risks and responsibility and live in a lower middle class environment for the next fifty years?"

4. *The second major trauma* and fatal wound of physicians in the progressive agenda on healthcare is that of preparing all physicians for maximal conscription into government controlled healthcare has now been accomplished with almost no possibility of reversal of the Affordable Care Act (ACA).

   The evidence of how well this agenda is working in 2014 was revealed in a media interview with Dr. Toby Cosgrove, CEO of the Cleveland Clinic healthcare system based in Cleveland, Ohio, on how the highly successful Cleveland Clinic medical system model was an ideal alternative outside of the ACA and government control.

   His affirmation that *58 percent of all doctors in the USA are now employed* by hospitals should only confirm that physicians are leaving private medical practice in excessive numbers. It further raises the question, "What is the root cause for this massive shift away from private medical practice to happen?"

   It's a complex problem that arose because of powerful political, social, and economic circumstances external to the practice of medicine.

   Because the professional practice of medicine is locked into the claws of government legally by licensure, appointed medical boards, and state laws, the practice of medicine has now become an indentured servant and plaything to be whipped into compliance by changing rules at every turn.

Unfortunately, the *practice of medicine is being divided* into segments, each of which salutes a different flag. It by no means requires that private medical practice must disappear. The ways to successfully retain private medical practice are what this treatise is all about.

"The cause of man's problem is lack of knowledge.
It does not stem from a shortage of information,
But rather from rejection of information."
-Hosea 4:6

The primary reasons why physicians are shifting away from private medical practice are simple and instructive:

1. Physicians and their medical practices are financially failing in increasing numbers. To survive, they sell their practices to hospitals and continue their medical practices under the control of the hospitals as employees.

2. To be able to make payments on their educational indebtedness, a significant source of income beginning promptly after graduation is required.

   Being essentially flat broke on graduation from medical school, what better option is available to them than to become employed with a reliable income source right from the start?

The fact remains:

There is a very reliable solution to almost all of physician's financial woes just sitting there waiting for implementation. Everyone in the business world knows what that solution is. And that's why every medical doctor's financial prowess for decades has been the laughingstock of the non-medical business profession.

The shame of it is that this lack of business education being taught can be reversed rather rapidly and the medical educators know it and do nothing to fix it.

The business education of all medical school students should *not be* an elective course. It's a fundamental knowledge required for every physician to reach their optimal value to patients, themselves, and our nation.

5. When you add extreme educational debts to the already over-the-top factors that are causing such pervasive frustration among private practice physicians, you get the seeds of destruction of medical professionals, the quality of medical care, and the future of healthcare. Substitution of "physician" by the term "healthcare provider" leaves no doubts about the true future of the profession.

6. *Over half of graduating medical students* today are headed into employed positions, understandably, because of the punishing education debts that need to be paid, starting about a year from graduation. This is not a voluntary choice for most new doctors who have finally confronted the reality of the power of money, theirs and others.

   By segmenting physicians into categories, *private practice verses employed doctors,* the pendulum now swings over to the side of all physicians who are employed by, or otherwise indentured to, a higher authority, like physicians in academic medicine, research, or administrative positions.

   It means that the indentured physicians have become "satisfied" with their position, voluntary or not, as one would expect. They are, at least to some degree, then vulnerable to the "statist's" (a designation given to progressives by Mark R. Levin in his new book, *Liberty and Tyranny)* subliminal brainwashing.

   When you live in their house, you can't help but eventually believe as they do for lack of another experience comparison and your comfort zone is established within that experience (ex. Patty Hearst kidnap case).

D. **The universal battle against medical practice restrictions.**

The daily mental distress that most medical doctors, who practice in the managed care model and are expected to live and practice with, can occur only because every single doctor is inherently adaptable at heart. It stems from a personality trait all physicians seem to possess: an entrepreneurial spirit. Their passion for practicing medicine includes the freedom to control their own medical career path and destiny—and is prevented from doing so when they are being controlled.

John G. Freymann, MD, head of the National Fund for Medical Education, expressed the critical issue concerning the need for a business education of doctors, as follows:

"If future physicians were introduced to economic reality, the medical profession might cease to be part of the cost problem and become part of the solution."
-John G. Freymann, MD,

So far, his nudging has not succeeded in persuading anyone, physicians or medical school academics, to follow his studied advice.

And it's my admonition exactly: to keep on nudging for business-trained physicians even more.

It's the right thing to do for hundreds of reasons.

3. Lack of tort reform regarding medical malpractice consequences

Every physician understands that almost every physician in the practice of medicine does so knowing that the probability of facing medical malpractice litigation sometime in their career is likely. During a long career in practice, it's expected.

Learning how to avoid a medical malpractice suit is not taught during a doctor's medical education. The knowledge is assimilated intermittently through conversations, reading materials one stumbles upon, occasional lectures offered at meetings, and from true stories about what happened to other doctors who were caught in the malpractice trap.

Physicians are especially vulnerable for many reasons. Most can handle the occurrence when it happens to them, but it leaves hidden scars in everyone that add up over time.

The problem of medical malpractice and its effect on the lives and careers of physicians is unpredictable and often devastating. Medical careers can end suddenly after only one incident. Physicians can easily lose everything they have, including family, reputation, and material holdings.

Those are traumatic events that never leave the minds of physicians who go through the ordeal. By definition it becomes a source of PTSD syndrome (post-traumatic stress disorder) for physicians to recover from if they can.

Clearly, the malpractice gauntlet is both a lesson and a punishment that may keep recurring. This brings up the issue of punishment without cause.

Frivolous malpractice legal actions are endemic with no end in sight. Even when the physician is found innocent of malpractice charges or allegations, they are under suspicion in the medical community, put through an unnecessary legal process such as hospital medical staff restrictions, and add another mental scar to the pile.

These are risks all doctors in medical practice accept or they wouldn't enter medical practice. Doctors accept the fact that they may make medical treatment mistakes for which a penalty applies. When they make a terrible mistake from bad judgment or actions, they punish themselves even more than is required by law.

Some quit practicing. Some completely change the way they practice and some are able to compensate for the mistake and continue practicing, but it never leaves their mind.

Beyond all these risk expectations is another world of hurt that remains in full force and without end.

Remember that the survival of every physician in these drastic malpractice cases also takes a huge financial toll on them. With a sound business education at least they are able to recover better than those who lack that education.

These reasons are why medical malpractice creates a strong and increasing desire to quit medical practice and the medical profession itself.

1. **Medical malpractice** is an unrelenting risk to all physicians in medical practice, with no expectation that there will be any legal relief from the risk in the near future, if ever.

The fact that *about six states* (as of this date) have in the past passed laws to cap the jury verdicts and awards concerning the *pain and suffering* element of a malpractice award, establishes the extent to which malpractice law affects the lives of nearly all physicians.

That's because these states decided to keep their doctors practicing there rather than causing them to move to another state where physicians are better protected. About thirty-one states have some sort of legal "capping" process (and that is a stretch) in place.

The fact that the *remaining forty-six states* have not passed the same protective liability laws and statutes over the last thirty or so years in our country, validates the power and influence that the *trial lawyer lobby* has. After all, it's not politically acceptable to destroy the cash cow these lawyers need to survive, right? So the battle continues.

Remember, lawyers dominate nearly all legislative bodies in our country and they are not about to vote for capping malpractice cases.

As recently as March 14, 2014, the *Wall Street Journal* reported that the *Florida Supreme Court declared that caps on medical malpractice verdicts were unconstitutional.* You can expect more problems from this for medical doctors.

In 2003 Jeb Bush, then governor, signed the law to keep doctors from leaving Florida because of unlimited jury verdicts that were causing a flood of doctors to leave Florida to practice elsewhere. The same problem has occurred in Nevada and Pennsylvania more recently.

2. **Malpractice cases do destroy medical practices and doctors.**

Doctors know that there will be unintentional mistakes made during their careers. They also know that a *single mistake* in judgment while treating patients can destroy their career and their family.

Because these errors occur unexpectedly and unintentionally, every physician throughout their careers fears losing everything they have worked and studied hard for.

Doctors in the high-risk medical specialties are most vulnerable and subject to greater fear. It's why doctors quit obstetrics and orthopedic surgeons resort to safer surgical procedures.

Medical malpractice risk consequently results in more restrictive practice of medicine. It leads to less medical practice income as well as financially threatens the careers of so many doctors.

A business education provides the tools for survival from medical malpractice litigation catastrophes and adds hope to doctors in this situation. They know they can start over again and know how to do it rather than suffer the hopelessness that normally follows these cases.

Note: (Wall Street Journal, March 29, 2014)
An article concerning California's new approach to elevating the CAP amount placed in 1975 of $250,000 on the pain and suffering "segment" of the Medical Malpractice Law, to a *$1,000,000 or more.*

It originated over one case involving death of two children in an automobile wreck caused by a medical patient who overdosed on *prescription* medication.

The proposal is to require medical professionals to check prescription drug histories of patients against a state pharmacy drug dispensed database (another egregious requirement of a doctor's time).

In essence, doctors would end up footing the bill for damage done by their own medical patients for which doctors are not liable. The cost of malpractice premiums will go up again—and physicians are punished as a scapegoat even more.

The case originated from the father of the children after the settlement in favor of the parents was considered by the parents inadequate when the father said his children were worth a lot more money than what they received.

It would seem now that there is a new standard being established for the monetary value of a child killed in an auto accident. In addition, medical doctors will become defendants in legal cases involving their own medical patients. Patients who abuse prescription medications and who end up in court as a result, means that prosecutors will certainly include the physicians who prescribed the medication, further increasing legal risks of practicing doctors.

The legal process also may well become a politically legal manipulation of the medical malpractice law guidelines to establish an additional method of acquiring that increased amount of money from a physician's insurance. Physicians legally and ethically have no known liability whatsoever in my view related to control of their patients actions (driver of the car: defendant) or the automobile accident she was responsible for.

Attorneys dominate the legislatures, so why not legally create a law revision to further pad their wallets?

3. Malpractice punishment goes far beyond the courtroom.

The punishment that any physician may experience as the aftermath of medical malpractice litigation strikes even deeper into the flesh. *Medical boards can punish physicians regardless of the litigation outcome* when circumstances indicate and their mood is favorable. Criteria for punishment are variable and often being highly subjective in nature.

Any doctor who takes the time to read the law statutes that pertain to the practice of medicine in the state where they are licensed can readily understand how soft the laws are concerning the interpretation of the laws by the courts and the medical boards. Have the medical academic scholars read the law?

If they did, or do read the laws pertaining to such legal statutes, they may recognize another reason or two why physicians might need the backup of an academic business education to help finance their increased malpractice premium.

Medical boards are composed of doctors and other civilians (all appointed and directly responsible to the governor) who make their decisions about doctor's actions based upon their interpretation of what the law seems to indicate to them. The process of a board's judgment and penalty of any doctor's crime or infraction is entirely subjective in nature. The seriousness of the infraction of the law is open to wide interpretation by each member of the board.

To my knowledge, there is no legal list within any state statutes that specify a certain punishment for each possible medical board infraction.

The punishment for each physician's "crime" is made by evaluation, investigation, discussion, and a vote by board members.

That's why the final vote can be so easily swayed by a loud and demanding pronouncement by a board member against a physician, which intimidates others on the board to agree with them. I have personally witnessed such an occurrence and it's a compelling reason to have your lawyer present any time you face a medical board for any reason.

An actual medical board case: biased and highly subjective.

A medical board case like this occurred in Arizona several years ago. It involved an OBG doctor who had applied for medical practice licensure there. He had been in OBG private medical practice at that time for over fifteen years and another eight years prior to that as a military doctor and resident in training, with only two malpractice cases (one settled and another he won in court). He had trained at an elite residency program in Philadelphia under a well-known academic medical education professor (who was a credentialed OBG board examiner).

A year prior to this, he had decided to leave the state he was practicing in for financial reasons and because of a third malpractice case where he had unintentionally made a bad medical judgment about an OB case and was the first time that it had ever happened. There were many contributing issues on the doctor's side that were totally ignored by the board: divorce litigation, bankruptcy, and financial problems with his practice.

The medical board reviewed his medical licensure history and questioned everything. All except one of the board members were satisfied with his qualifications for unrestricted licensure. One younger OBG female doctor and member of the board was loudly persistent in her criticism of his bad judgment in his last malpractice case while using every descriptive means to describe how incompetent he was in her estimation.

It was not because of his obstetrical delivery competence, but because of his bad judgment he made in this one single case over all the twenty-three years he had practiced quality medicine.

Finally, she was able to convince the minds of all the other "non-OB doctors" on the panel who were forced to take her word about the judgment issues. They could have obtained another OBG consultant's opinion of the doctor's actions to rule out the personal prejudice of this OBG doctor on the board which was very obvious, but didn't. There were other alternatives available, but not taken.

In this case, the medical board could have required supervision of this doctor in obstetrics for a reasonable period of time (usually six months to a year) and granted full licensure—and didn't.

What do other specialists really know themselves about acceptable management of OB cases?

Not granting full licensure in obstetrics and gynecology becomes a permanent black mark on this doctor's records. One biased decision by the medical board permanently obstructs the rest of any doctor's career and financial status. It may prevent other state medical licensures or result in severe limitations on a licensure because those records are made available to all USA state medical boards and other pertinent legal agencies when requested.

His prior OB management of obstetrical cases over the prior fifteen years was by all standards exemplary. This was a clear example of how a biased board member (regardless of what the bias origin was) can sway the whole panel's decision making. The doctor was granted a "gyn-only" practice licensure after a long deliberation of the case by the medical board.

This was another example of how important it is for a physician to have his own attorney during any medical board interaction, but this doctor didn't think of that and assumed his credentials spoke for themselves.

Many of the judgments made by the medical boards are whims of their personal biases, therefore unpredictable. Punishments by medical boards may include being required to undergo a residency training over again after being in flawless OBG practice for many years: imagine the cost and economic hardship on a doctor and his family forced to do a repeat residency after all those years of trouble free medical practice.

Today such a punishment would financially cripple any medical doctor, his or her ambition, family relationships, and likely would create debt that one could never recover from, let alone all the associated catastrophes associated with this situation.

Self-punishment

If you don't have the money to make it through the required repeat residency, then you would be forced to quit medical practice, change careers, try to apply for licensure in another state, find a new wife, or contemplate suicide by immolation or other means. The self-punishment can be fatal and, unfortunately, does sometimes happen.

This happens primarily because a doctor prepares for only one career in medicine. They are not prepared for any other career should the need arise. When their medical career ends involuntarily, finding another occupation is a major problem, takes a long time, and with no income source readily available, life becomes hopeless rapidly.

Any physician who inadvertently causes harm to a patient, or unintentionally is involved in such an event, yet accused, will always have the event fixed so firmly in their mind that the memory of that self-induced guilt will continue to shadow them for the rest of their lives. They often never forgive themselves for not being perfect.

Unintentional injuries to patients, when severe, often force doctors to make major changes in their medical practice functions and focus. Bad obstetrical delivery cases often lead doctors to severely limit their future OB care or quit doing obstetrics altogether.

Many of these cases should never force doctors into such unnecessary alterations of their practice, but they do. Doctors are quick to judge themselves much more critically than is reasonable in the eyes of their peers.

The effects of this self-induced punishment often lead to mental problems like loss of self-esteem, uncertainty about their own competence, fear that they might perform other unintentional bad deeds as well, and often significantly reduces their passion to practice medicine at all.

By funneling their practice down to lower-risk patients, they lose income and don't know how to market their practice to bring their income back up again.

The family punishment

The sudden drop in medical practice income often ignites family conflicts. Divorce happens often. Why would a wife stick around when her husband loses his medical license and no longer can support the family?

Once a physician's practice is disrupted by a malpractice case being filed, his or her mind normally begins to insert doubt about thinking clearly. That may lead to him or her becoming very withdrawn from family, friends, and social interaction. Communications decrease. Spouses are kept out of the picture. Time with the family is reduced.

More time is spent at the office in an effort to improve practice income that may occur later, planning for the worst outcome, seeking advice from close friends, making decisions about "what if… situations."

Bad moods are commonly occur, and the family may just stay away from the doctor, even the office staff as well. Family members have no idea how to react to the parent-doctor, so they avoid everything that isn't necessary. This leads the family into turmoil about what's going to happen next and if they will ever get back to normal again.

The problem with this situation is that getting credible help, counseling, and advice almost always comes late in the picture—even too late.

Drug and alcohol use complicates everything and family life often continues to disintegrate, especially if addiction treatment is required for the doctor. A high school friend (physician) of mine in general practice became addicted to drugs, lost his family and practice, and was able and allowed to practice only in a hospital under the watchful eye of his peers for many years after.

The hospital staff punishment

The hospital staff may also initiate supervision of the physician for a period of time to ensure the doctor's medical staff privileges are appropriate and no further problems occur. Such factors may result in restricted hospital privileges and immediate loss of patient admission privileges.

If a doctor happens to already be on staff at other hospitals, he can admit his patients to those hospitals. But for doctors practicing in an area where there is only one hospital and this happens, it essentially will often destroy his medical practice.

When a doctor's medical staff privileges are restricted, it must be reported to the state medical board and becomes a permanent black mark on a doctor's medical practice record at the state medical board. It's also available to other state medical boards forever. When you later try to get a medical license in another state, the issue is plastered across the first page of the report they ask for.

When a doctor doesn't have close friends on hospital committees, it creates far more practice problems. Peers often have biases towards other doctors. They tend to vote in hospital medical committees against a doctor, or his ideas and beliefs, and who they already dislike because of trouble outside the hospital environment.

Doctor friends on the committees, who know your quality, personal character, medical skills, and integrity, are the ones who influence decisions about you and speak on your behalf in a positive way.

Being put on supervision or probation is not required to be reported to medical boards under usual circumstances. Probation and supervision can be altered over time and removed when there is evidence that the problem will not be repeated.

Doctors, who never have much contact with you, learn about your real attributes, integrity, and competence during committee functions.

A malpractice case, its ramifications, and jury judgments made against a hospital staff member is a threat to any hospital as well as to the hospital staff. The threat to the hospital is that it may be included in the judgment, cost the hospital millions of dollars, or even shut it down.

The threat to the medical staff is dependent on whether the hospital where they all practice in is put out of business as a result of the severe penalty that the court applies to it financially, often because they allowed this bad doctor on to their medical staff.

Severe malpractice cases judged against you, whether fair or not, whether warranted or not, are perceived by medical staffs and your peers as a doctor being guilty and responsible at least to some extent. That prompts most medical staffs to investigate you, evaluate you (no matter how long they have known you or the reputation you had prior), and are forced into some kind of punishment of you just to maintain hospital standards and bylaws.

The medical community punishment

In the local medical community all problems of doctors become widely known faster than a speeding bullet. A major consequence for most doctors is that they no longer get patient referrals or requests for consultations.

Socially, they may often feel the sting. Good friends become distant.

These matters can't be resolved by a business education, but it certainly enables a physician the leverage to recover faster and more effectively financially—and *that may be even more important* than all the rest put together.

One consolation is that if perspective medical students find out about all these risks, they probably wouldn't believe them anyway. If students really understood all the risks and believed they were true, many probably would avoid or quit medical school today.

4. Why the lack of useable and effective business knowledge is always the stalking enemy of every private practicing physician.

Almost all graduating medical students today have little or no formal or experiential business education save the incidental and intermittent fragments of information about business gathered from parents, college economic courses, part time jobs, or fathers who are physicians and share their practice business experiences with them.

This regrettable consequence is destined to directly interfere with the goals of nearly all medical doctors. For some doctors it will actually destroy the medical practice financial future of their careers.

The usual fallible resource about how a private medical practice can be set up that is commonly used by over 95 percent of medical doctors is an accumulation of business advice from other local practicing doctors, information and advice from other medical practice office staffs, practice management literature about medical practice business and the employees you hire at the beginning.

The consequence of this approach sets the stage for practice business chaos and continued loss of practice income during their medical career.

It gives rise to the most fundamental cause for financial failure of medical practices, both now and previously, and immediately surfaces in the minds of rational thinking individuals.

The sad part about this becomes evident when physicians years later begin to recognize how much more efficient, productive, and successful their practice would have been if they had understood and implemented business strategies and tools along the way that every successful commercial business uses.

The thrust of medical education should be to engage the minds of physicians while they are already in the "learning mode" while in medical school.

It bears repeating that years of medical practice history have documented that rarely do physicians, after finishing medical school and further specialty training, decide to set aside time to take on any aspect of a formal business education. It's true even when they understand how much it would help their existing or future medical practice business.

That's the reason it has to be done while in medical school when their minds are ready to accept it.

5. Every physician's discovery that reaching their original professional goals will be impossible

Those rare physicians who subsequently do reach their ultimate goals in medical practice are not prepared to admit that their success was the result of contributing factors beyond the scope of their own personal talents, skills, and business knowledge.

Everyone knows that wealthy families, for example, can and often do provide the finances necessary for their son or daughter to overcome any and all barriers to their ultimate medical practice goals one way or another. Thus, it lends credence to the value of having a formal business education that permits all physicians to make the level of income necessary to do the same.

Thank God that there are physicians who have personal and career goals that don't require such a strong need to climb the ladder as high as some do. But even for those physicians goals change, circumstances change, and passions sometimes even increase along the way.

For these "less driven" physicians, there remains the same necessity for a formal business education whether they think they will use it or not. If a physician quits medical practice early and changes to another career, having a proficient knowledge of business is still a great advantage.

Many physicians today already realize that starting an outside business has practical and economic advantages that supplement their medical practice objectives. With a strong business education, that outside effort is much easier and more likely profitable.

Having an efficient, productive, and profitable medical practice, continues to be a major source of career satisfaction and fulfillment for every physician regardless of the variable objectives sought.

"The impact of money and income on physicians in private medical practice especially are undeniably related to the degree of success and ultimate quality and competence of virtually all physicians."

Debate about how much that the revenue from medical practice contributes to the satisfaction of every physician is useless—it's a fact!

Anyone who denies that the inadequate amount of money earned in medical practice today is not the primary cause of physician frustration is lacking in judgment and diligence.

Why then is a formal business education of medical students lacking in the medical curriculums of medical schools today? Please explain that to me, if you can.

6. Discovery by doctors that reaching their personal goals and obligations to their family will have to be downgraded.

For the majority of practicing physicians whose take-home incomes are progressively decreasing across a variety of specialties, their continued loyalty to the medical profession is rapidly declining.

Only after doctors have been exposed to investment grade business information and felt the sting of a financially failing medical practice, does reality set-in. They're in a professional business that has proven to them that the rewards are not nearly equivalent to those of many other professional and commercial businesses.

Financial freedom is not in the cards for most doctors as the profession exists today. When they see cardiac bypass surgeons suddenly without a job, obstetricians quitting obstetrics for fear of the malpractice risk, and the proliferation of employed "robotized" doctors being forced into employment servitude forever, doctors' options for survival are narrowing.

Truly, the impact of not being able to afford to send their kids to college and beyond, the inability to fund a retirement plan, and the necessity of their family living a lower middle-class existence will seriously extinguish any continued desire to try harder... in addition to putting more thought into leaving the profession.

The doctors themselves can usually learn to adapt to these sacrifices, but when it also significantly affects the welfare of their families, it pierces the heart of their integrity, professional purpose, and passion for their profession. That's a wound that doesn't heal.

You see, there are some *more important things* in life than the practice of medicine. One has only to look at the new-age generation of physicians' preference to work a nine-to-five shift and is not hesitant to drop off the care of their patients to others at the end of their shift, to understand the new trend.

So it seems, at least to older doctors, who never thought in terms of medical practice gauged by the clock, and who only thought in terms of responsibility to patients as being unrestricted by the clock.

Now, take those same new-age doctors, give them the business tools to make as much money as they choose, and they will remain satisfied, fulfilled, and happy in the practice of medicine. This I believe as strongly as I do the Bible commandments and the power of faith.

Give medical students a strong business education and they will outperform during their medical careers in extraordinary fashion. In addition, the benefits to the medical schools and universities will be far above the present-day rewards.

7. Expectations that doctors had for their medical careers, will *not* be reached.

Expectations create hope, extreme desire, and ongoing search for more information. Medical student memory of medical facts (and business principles) is shaped by expectations.

Students are often faced with information overload, which will be blocked out unless it is simple enough to understand and if they have enough time to process it.

According to Barbara E. Kahn, professor of Marketing at the Wharton School of Business, University of Pennsylvania, in her book, *Global Brand Power,* in which she presents the logical sequence of implementation of student expectations into the learning process (as adapted to medical education):

> *"Consideration of important factors is a function of a student's willingness to search for information. The amount of search is a function of an intuitive cost-benefit analysis. If a perceived benefit exists for taking the time and trouble to search for information, they will; if not, they stop at 'good enough.'*
>
> *When preconceived expectations do not exist, students will generally search more extensively before making a decision or choice.*
>
> *New collected information is interpreted alongside existing information. Students take the information they already think they know and tend to reject information that runs counter to preconceived ideas (called confirmation bias)."*

This learning sequence is clearly applicable to and explains why preconceived ideas and beliefs often strongly interfere with the acknowledgment that *business education plays a critical part* in every doctor's career capabilities, extent of success accomplishments, and maximal satisfaction with their medical practice and medical careers.

Unless there is a profound commitment by medical school teaching staff and educators to actually change the preconceived notion and past medical tradition posture that business education is not essential to a physician's success, then the medical education system is definitely contributing wholeheartedly and intentionally to the financial failure of physicians and their medical practices.

If medical school educators know the necessity and value of business knowledge to private practicing physicians, and then to continue to neglect the business education of physicians, it's intentional, abusive, and unforgivable.

Private practice physicians witness daily what a business education could do for their private medical practice—but it doesn't sink in. Every physician is eager to do better and to improve on their skills, medical knowledge, and practice revenue. The problem is that most have no idea about how to accomplish it.

The greatest difficulty is to try to overcome the static biases of the medical professional educational hierarchy, who may not know what they think they know.

The problem faced here is a long-standing one. For none of the stiff-necked contributors to the lack of a business education of physicians (and medical students) are willing to step out of their box and take responsibility, especially when the problem can be solved more easily and is less costly in the long run than they think. That reveals lack of diligence in medical education.

So what gives me the right to criticize and offer possible solutions? The fact that I am a living example of what that lack of a business education cost me in my medical career, which at the time I only had one option open to me, to watch my practice disappear while I looked on helplessly as the process unfolded.

Yes, there is much more to my story than simply being business ignorant and lacking the business tools I needed to at least give me a fighting chance to rescue my practice.

8. Lack of a business education has now become a co-conspirator and promoter of ethical slippage by providing the perfect stimulus for physicians to push the legal and ethical boundaries of private medical practice in order to survive in the medical profession

Believe it or not, agree with me or not, the mounting threats to every physician's medical career today are more dangerous than ever—dangerous because these threats have pushed physicians into survival tactics. Those tactics have created a widespread proliferation of evidence and real examples of borderline legal and ethical medical practice action, some even illegal and unethical by any standard.

Some of those tactics that private practice physicians consider necessary for their medical practice survival result in the destruction of physicians and their careers almost daily across this nation.

Such quasi-legal and ethical issues are widely publicized in the media, which adds another log to the fire of indignation felt by medical patients and the public in general towards the medical profession.

Cornered doctors will stretch the limits of their creative abilities to search out and use whatever tactics that seem to them the most effective means to protect themselves and their medical practices from financial ruin.

Face it—after over twenty-two years of educational preparation, over $200,000 to pay for a professional career, wouldn't you go to extremes to prevent losing it all, even if it had the potential for jail time?

Strategies for escaping from practice restrictions

Take the most recent published cases that serve to document what doctors are doing now to escape financial disaster and worse. An April 10, 2014 *Wall Street Journal* (and other media as well) article on the Medicare medical billings by various doctors around our nation does a lot more than let the public in on several methods doctors use to make money.

When a single medical doctor is able *to bill millions of dollars* to Medicare annually, it reflects poorly on other doctors, even if it may be perfectly legitimate billings from an ethical doctor. The issue does indicate that this issue is just the tip of the iceberg for thousands of other doctors doing the same thing on a smaller scale and in many other ways all done to maintain their practice income, family obligations, and lifestyle.

If you take a moment to consider the ramifications of these issues, you may clearly understand how a doctor *with a formal business education* in private medical practice can, and usually does, manage to recover financially, without having to resort to any quasi-legal tactics.

They have the business knowledge not only to prevent financial threats to their careers that cause the intensely driven emotion to "stretch the boundaries" beyond acceptable, but also to rescue their medical practice using business tools that are known to solve these situations when they occur.

You and I know that this problem will not go away and will predictably worsen if "business education" is not seared into the minds of medical students. Any doctor with a formal business education stored in their brain will be the last one standing in the end—no, not in front of the firing squad.

You also know that physicians resort to "code-cheating," overbilling, doing unnecessary surgical procedures, select higher paying medical procedure coding when there are less costly alternatives, multiple-visit billing instead of all done in one visit, referrals of medical patients to other doctors to assist at their patient's surgery, referrals of patients to doctors to perform surgery on their patients when surgery is not indicated, and many other examples resulting from being financially cornered.

All these slippery tactics are done for the most part because the doctors have no other means of survival—at least financially—and are without adequate business knowledge that could have avoided these issues.

Incredibly, these financially induced disasters can nearly all be resolved starting today if every medical student is provided with an academic business education along with their medical education.

The objectives, as I have said before, are to prevent doctors from losing their private medical practices and quitting medical practice. Preventing attrition and keeping medical doctors in practice much longer is equally important. When studies and statistics show that about 50 percent of female doctors practice only part-time, the necessity for providing a business education is tripled, at the very least.

Egregious implications that dishonor the medical profession

It's interesting to see and read about how large organizations and industries go about choosing how to spend their money and what to spend it on.

To that point, an interview with Roger Goodell, Commissioner of the National Football League, just before Super Bowl "48," included questions from Chris Wallace about what they are doing to protect the players from injuries. This $10 billion sports industry is now spending mega-millions of dollars on player's health and treatment of long term extensive injuries, like concussion brain injuries.

Medical evidence and surveys have documented the serious nature of brain concussions on the players, although some will argue that the action taken to improve the safety of the players was done to financially benefit the NFL coffers and line the pockets of the owners.

I submit to you that even if that is true to some extent, the benefits provided to the players, teams, and supportive people (including doctors) go much further and deeper into the decision making process to make the right and honorable changes that are warranted and necessary.

Medical schools should take away a lesson like this themselves.

This real example of just one industry's decision to spend a huge amount of money for the benefit of its players is no different than *a billion-dollar medical education system* providing financial support for the protection of the healthcare industry by providing *an academic business education* for all medical students today.

Being tactical about today is OK, but it's significantly better to be strategic about tomorrow.

Protection means that every medical student should be protected primarily against medical practice financial failure, but includes stimulation of personal familiar heuristics. Increasing frustration with medical practice (relating to and likely the cause for the attrition of most of the physicians today) can be resolved to a great degree *by providing an academic business education for all medical students.*

Is it too outrageous to assume that the highly intelligent academic medical school and medical profession scholars certainly know what's causing a severe degeneration of the private practice segment of the medical profession?

Everyone must understand that it's the lack of adequate income that is precipitating the frustration, disappointment, and attrition among physicians. If you don't believe that's the cause, then why is it that wealthy medical doctors rarely, if ever, are disappointed, frustrated, and leave the profession? (I've worked with a few of these wealthy physicians.)

Wake up!

Another significant point and lesson about the NFL example that one should consider is that of the *responsibility they feel for taking care of the problem.* It's voluntary. The administrators of the NFL are not financially required to do what they are doing, but it is the *right and moral thing to do.*

Are there any medical school educators, medical education scholars, or medical administrative CEOs out there reading this who feel even minimum responsibility for providing a formal business education for all medical students?

No, the medical school staff should not do the teaching. The medical school is responsible for providing it, not teaching it—using any means available.

In a similar sense, medical school academics can't be forced to add a business education to medical student curriculums. The *stimulus must be voluntary action* taken by education scholars because it is the ethical and moral thing to do, especially when all the evidence about this issue proves that *the students and physicians will not do this of their own volition.*

Because medical school educators cleverly transfer that responsibility to the students and physicians alike, it reflects on their belief that such a determination is completely acceptable and honorable.

To continue to stand by and watch the results of letting the medical doctors suffer the indignities, humiliating affronts, and insulting and disgraceful injuries accompanying their lack of essential medical business knowledge, is irresponsible and unacceptable.

Furthermore, because the medical school curriculum hierarchy has done absolutely nothing of significance to resolve this tragedy over the last century, their complacency will continue to be the standard for the future, unless this irresponsible activity by medical educators is exposed. This group of medical educators believe that their distinguished efforts in educating the most competent and intelligent physicians in the world today is enough, but it's not!

Sir Winston Churchill made a very appropriate statement when he said, *"It's not enough that we do our best; sometimes we have to do what's required."*

What has actually happened in the medical education field is that the well deserved accolades medical educators remain so proud of, is the camouflage that hides their unforgivable lack of responsibility to comply with what is necessary: an academic business education of all medical students.

There are many more examples of doing the right thing.

Football-players earn enough money to pay cash for all their own medical injuries and even go so far as to sign a contract that clearly spells out the dangers and increased risks associated with playing professional football. But they accept and are legally responsible for their own health problems and injuries, assuming that health insurance in not considered in this circumstance.

In the same sense, don't medical education academics have a responsibility to take action to resolve a problem that they clearly see resulting from doctors who lack a business education?

At least, don't academic scholars have a moral and ethical responsibility to do something about the deficiency, especially when they are in the right position at the right time, to resolve the business education problem?

If you haven't really thought about it, let me inform you…

This is a desperate medical school education crisis of unlimited proportions that must be faced and fixed today!

"A lot of things are black and white and we create ever widening gray areas between them because we lack the courage required by clarity and truth."
-Dan S. Kennedy

We are in an odyssey of generational academic indifference towards the business side of private medical practice, and it's a self-destructive position that must be changed.

(Review, with a different slant)

Prior to 1960 fee for service in the practice of medicine had become the healthcare environment that made the medical profession desirable and attractive as a career.

Most medical students at that time understood that a physician had the freedom to treat medical patients in their own manner unhindered by forces outside of medicine. This exploded their desire to go as far up the medical practice success ladder as they desired during their medical careers.

This upward momentum was not only possible, but affordable for most. It was supported by a rapid escalation of medical technology. Better medical care was the result and no one complained. *During the 1960s* the costs of medical care increased dramatically, but were accepted in light of better medical care.

Older doctors today remember this era of physicians being blamed for the escalating costs of healthcare all too well.

Doctors became the scapegoats for the rising healthcare costs when in fact medical technology and innovation sparked an overwhelming demand by patients for physicians to apply the new technology whether the patient needed it or not. All pregnant women wanted an ultrasound to see their fetus on the screen, for example. If their doctor didn't do that procedure, the patient would find one that did.

It became the start of a new generation of patients who demanded services and doctors were obliged to comply with patient demands or lose patients and income. *Doctors were not the cause of rising healthcare costs!*

By the early 1970s the managed care systems were born with the anointing of the government and large labor unions. This short and sketchy history reminds us of what has happened and changed in medical practice and healthcare over the last five decades.

The real turning point for physicians began about 1970. At that time physicians in private practice were losing a large percentage of their patients to the various managed care healthcare facilities. This began the gradual decline in private medical practice revenue.

The later increase of practice guidelines, practice fee restrictions, and control of healthcare in many ways has added another millstone to the work for medical practice income.

By the 1980s, the significant reduction in medical doctor incomes became permanent and has been declining since. This means that physicians in general had been placed in a position where physicians could not do much of anything to increase their incomes, other than working harder and seeing more patients.

There are *two primary causes* why innumerable physicians today are being forced out of private medical practice and hundreds out of their medical careers.

1. Physicians have never been taught how to efficiently and profitably manage the business of medical practice—and never were provided a formal business education (including marketing).

2. Physicians have never been taught how to use business and marketing tools proven to keep them out of financial quicksand in the first place. The ultimate result is that *the business of medicine* has been cleverly and intentionally hidden from the ears and minds of all medical students to the point that they "don't know what they don't know" and the world of business escapes their thinking.

No Business Education + No Business Tools = Business Failure

CHAPTER 4

The Wound

"Lack of Business Education Accountability Undermines Every Physician's Full Potential and Violates the Career and Professional Responsibility of Every Medical School's Education Commitment"

Conscience is sufficient grounds for condemnation because it establishes a framework of right and wrong and reflects the real truth written in their hearts and minds.

RESPONSIBILITY AND ACCOUNTABILITY are commonly held to be essential ingredients of medical school education. However, the extent to which they are used, who's responsible, and the boundaries ascribed to their application, remain nebulous. This is where the debate begins.

Although medical educators may have legitimate reasons for dismissing their obligation to provide a formal business education for all medical students, there remains the responsibility of educators to provide a "complete" education of medical students to the best of their ability.

Many medical school educators are convinced that the responsibility for a business education lies only with the medical student or doctor at some later time.

When one factors in the present-day instability of our economy, increasing governmental restrictions on healthcare provider fees, and the devastating effects of the ACA problems, epic financial problems of doctors follow. Those problems continue to be unresolved.

Anyone can see the valid reasons why even the most fixed-minded educational scholars find themselves having great difficulty rationalizing their objections to accepting any responsibility for providing a formal business education for all medical students.

Their reasons for refusing to provide this profoundly necessary business education no longer hold water today because:

- Physicians/students will not voluntarily ever go get a business education. This fact has shown to be documented over the last four decades.

- Physicians early in their career in medical practice will not go back to business school, take two years off medical practice with no other income available. They can't afford the $50,000 cost of a two-year MBA program when they are already being forced to start paying back their huge educational debts after they have graduated from medical school. It would on average add up to a debt of nearly $250,000 for most students, which inevitably would take over twenty years in medical practice to pay back while living frugally.

- As tuition continues to rise, only students from wealthy families will be able to afford a medical education, perhaps even a college education. Are medical schools prepared to resolve this issue by providing the discretionary funds to enable medical students to attend? I don't think so because government handouts to academic education are drying up. The logical end to this stretch is a catastrophe. It would not be a surprise if the process of future medical education goes back to an apprenticeship process known from ancient times.

- Any refusal of medical education scholars to accept responsibility for providing the business education of all medical students would clearly amount to an affirmation that…

    * It is perfectly reasonable in their minds that keeping the educational system as it is presently provided is acceptable.

* Accepting the business ignorance of physicians and the effects it has on the financial tragedies that happen to a majority of physicians in private medical practice today is a perfectly proper stand to hold to.

* The business side of medical practice was never meant to be learned, or taught, or of any reasonable value to physicians.

* Actually adding a formal business education into the regular medical school curriculum would not be possible, would be too difficult to do, would definitely interfere with the full medical curriculum, and would cost too much money to implement.

* There is no reason to do anything else that would definitely improve the knowledge and skills of physicians, would provide physicians a set of business skills that would certainly increase their career potential and enable them to create a medical practice business protected against financial failure.

As incredible as it seems, it is more than likely that these beliefs must have been, and still are, held by medical school education scholars for decades, if not centuries. Keeping the business education and business tools away from medical students should be a crime, in my opinion.

This presumes that academic medical school scholars neither care if the doctor financially fails in private medical practice, nor do they accept any obligation or responsibility to provide medical students with a business education.

Even when they know that the essential monetary rewards and benefits to physicians and the benefits to all future medical patients under their care are absolutely essential for the maintenance, growth, and profitably of their medical practices, they persist in their beliefs.

Why would the medical education academics do that?

One would normally expect that scholars of this elite caliber would recognize what would be the right thing to do and do it. But they don't, at least not yet.

Of course, there can be other ulterior motives among medical academic scholars that bind them to their fixed mindset. If the motive was pride in the quality of doctors they send out into the communities, then they should be shamefully reevaluating their personal self-aggrandizement involved with that motivation.

However, it isn't likely that a pride motivation is the basis for their thinking. The fact that medical school academics continue to graduate *business-ignorant* physicians that are predestined to fail financially, indicates that their thinking is shallow, their commitments unrealistic, and their obligations border on spurious.

In reality, these incredibly intelligent, skilled, and knowledgeable physicians in the care and treatment of medical patients are never provided with the business opportunity to use that extraordinary education to its maximum and optimal extent possible. What a shame it is that that situation exists today at a time when physicians deserve a business education the most as medical practice financial failures increase.

Maybe, medical academics think that medical students already understand everything about what an academic business education offers them? If so, that's errant optimism. Most all medical students enter medical school with absolutely no academic business education. When medical students don't know what they don't know, how will they ever discover that they truly need and must have a business education to reach their optimal potential in medical practice?

You already know the answer, right?

Medical education, lacking a companion business education, is often catapulted into recognition the minute that a physician can't pay the bills. It usually happens when a physician finally accepts the fact that his practice can no longer keep up with office expenses. At this point he's forced to overcome his denial that all was going OK.

He realizes that his patient load is actually disappearing. There's not enough money left-over even to pay for the business education that would allow him or her to recover from the disaster. I've been there and no physician should ever have to be confronted by such a catastrophic crossroads of complete hopelessness.

On the other side are the academic scholars who understand the importance of a formal business education, but for some reason don't do anything to make it happen. The following reasons seem to be the most obvious reasons why it never gets done.

Accountability for the business education of medical students is complex and yet amenable to sound reasoning and resolution among those who acknowledge the impact it has on medical practice and physician careers.

1. Are medical school professors and instructors not capable teachers of business knowledge? Then what?

Nearly all medical school educators have never themselves received a full academic business education, *so how can they teach it?*

The lack of their own business education is the most important reason why medical school professors aren't the best business teachers. It's one thing that helps guarantee that an optimal medical career success often escapes the minds of many of those who teach medical students.

Maybe you've noticed that those who make the most money in any profession are *not always* the smartest, most talented, or most experienced. In fact, sometimes they're downright ordinary!

So how is it that they figure out how to make so much money in medical practice and the rest of us never do? It's not because of the extensive amount of medical knowledge being stuffed into their brains, which is the necessary fuel that runs their medical business.

It's the ability to use their medical talents and expertise most effectively and productively (making money) and is the result of *knowing marketing strategies and knowing good business management.*

How do you invade the medical student's minds to change the preconceived thought that business knowledge isn't important to their careers or medical practice, which is the circumstance today?

The scholarly step-wise process is well known, but is rarely used in teaching medical students.

The recognized steps to learning anything:

a. *Knowledge is essential to belief.* When business knowledge is withheld from medical students, how could they believe?

b. *Real belief must be preceded by faith and confidence in the lesson being taught.* How do medical students gain faith and confidence in the pursuit of a business education if they have no idea what a business education can do for them?

c. *Faith must be preceded by hearing and/or seeing the essence of the lesson.* It means that the purpose and objectives of business strategies and tools must be explained to students.

d. *Hearing requires a knowledgeable teacher.* It's why medical school academics without a formal business education are not qualified to teach business. Business experts are.

Comment: There is ample evidence within the business community of a significant disparage between business schools usability of education (MBA degree) taught by business professors and the practical usability of a business education taught by entrepreneurial business experts who have been there and done it all.

Because this author has been educated in business by the latter group of business experts (most are multimillionaires) who have learned both from their own business experiences and the large number of other experts advice, I recommend this resource for learning business and marketing.

If you have ever interviewed medical students who had an MBA degree before entering medical school, you would quickly become aware that what these experts teach doctors far surpasses the usefulness and effectiveness of their MBA education.

In addition, by learning from the educational materials these experts make available to everyone, and are continuously updated, it's not difficult for anyone to become business-knowledgeable while sitting in your easy chair at home.

The cost of that education, depending on how deep you go to learn about business management and marketing, will normally range from under $5,000 (just buying and reading business books and digital educational products of the experts) to $25,000 (attending live seminars, workshops, and training events).

One can reasonably make a case that medical school teachers and instructors don't have adequate business knowledge to teach business principles and strategies. In addition, they are not fully educated in the teaching formats and educational processes used by students to learn things. This indicates that business should not be taught by medical professors and instructors. (See chapter 8 for details how this process can be handled.)

"One cannot teach what one does not live"
-James 3:13

However, there is at least one essential duty that the teaching professors and instructors are responsible for. Someone must speak out so that the medical students can hear from authoritative people about the necessity of a business education.

Students hearing the actual truthful testimonials have good reason to alter their negative preconceptions they previously assumed about business education for doctors. Once they hear it from the right teachers using the right persuasive language, then they usually will believe it. Otherwise, students who don't hear about why and how business knowledge helps their careers continue to disregard business knowledge as being essential to them and their medical careers.

It's doubtful that any business teachers would refuse to respond to such an easy task, if they were asked to do so.

How business education can best be provided to medical students is discussed later in this book (chapters 7 and 8).

2. Today most medical educators feel that the full responsibility lies with the medical students themselves, to obtain a business education if they choose.

To think that medical students are different, unique, or otherwise above or beyond reach for adapting to the additional formal business education during their medical school education is nothing more than academic self-sabotage.

Mastery of *medical business education* supremacy is enormously valuable and therefore requires disciplined study, patience, constant skill improvement, and creative application.

The belief by medical educators that they have no responsibility for providing a business education to medical students is the dominant belief nationwide today. If not, then why isn't it being done in at least one medical school today?

The case can be made reasonably that every medical student has up to now been responsible for all their own decisions they have made to this point in their career education. Why should all medical students not also be responsible to provide for their own business education by any means available?

The answer is yes, at least when the business education process occurs during their medical school education. The process has to be subjected to the factors that allow for sharing of their medical education time and learning responsibilities.

Both major benefits demand the need to be compatible. Medical schools have the desire to educate their doctor graduates to be the best in every category of medicine. So why not also be best in *the business of medical practice* as well?

Young doctors and upcoming medical students have the desire to learn everything possible that will advance their medical practice and career to a higher level than the average, even much higher.

The key is that a student's memory for both business principles and medical facts is shaped by their expectations. Their information overload issue will not be blocked out unless the information is simple enough to understand and if students have enough time to process it.

There are multiple reasons why medical students should not be held responsible for their own business education:

a. Medical students for the most part *have no idea about what they will need to know about medical practice business beforehand.* What would they study? Only after years in medical practice do they eventually recognize and accept that business knowledge would have helped their careers enormously, hence the need for a business education being taught while still in medical school.

b. Medical students have such a heavy medical education load, *there's no room for a business education course* as well. Many medical students have jobs, do research outside the school curriculum to earn money; those extracurricular projects document the fact that they actually do have time for outside things.

It gets down to how productively they use their time. When one researches this issue, the rationed and available time can be used much more effectively. It's a matter of having the self-discipline to prioritize the use of their time.

Medical schools *do* have plenty of room and time for providing a formal business education of students. Creative minds know that.

Another aspect of medical schools having "curricular room" for a business education course can be legitimized by deleting the very superficial medical courses that schools have been added to medical education and which are later useful only to very few doctors.

Again, that also is a matter of the school's priority of educational importance.

c. Medical students are apt to *avoid a business education course even if it is provided to them and voluntary.* One thing that routinely happens regarding medical students actions during medical school that counters this argument, is the power and fear of "losing out" on something important being offered to a limited few students.

A very good example of this happened during my first year as a medical student. Over half of the class flat-out flunked the final exam in Biochemistry.

The teaching staff sensed that their instructive messages had not been delivered in a memorable manner. Before providing a re-examination for the medical class, those that did not pass the test were instructed to attend a few evening classes to review the biochemistry course information.

To the surprise of everyone and after all the failing students were seated, the remaining segment of the class that had already passed the test showed up and filled up the standing room along the classroom walls.

It is a convincing argument that the fear of letting other classmates get ahead of them by leaving themselves out of the picture was not only unacceptable, but also would never happen whatever the barriers were.

This example illustrates what would likely happen should any formal business course series be offered on a *voluntary* participation basis. All the class would also commit to the same objective for fear of losing a rare opportunity that would be of remarkable benefit to them later.

The advantage of such a business course being *required* instead of voluntary upgrades the importance and value of the course in the eyes of the students.

This effect is also found as a marketing strategy. For example, when one gets a book on an interesting topic for free and a book on the same topic is sold for $25, the perception is that the $25 book contains much more value to the buyer. And when the book costs $95, it certainly must have considerably more value than a $25 one. Perception must be dealt with and is not always correct.

d. *Creating a formal business course for medical students is not affordable.* This concern may be another barrier to establishing such a valuable business education.

There are many options available to smash any worry about affordability. When a medical school spends $18 million or so on a new building on campus for some special purpose that already has a place that they have been using to work in, certainly makes a campus look nicer, but may not be absolutely necessary at that time or in the long run.

The cost of adding a new course or curriculum to the medical school curriculum is nowhere near as much as adding a new building. And the value and profitability of such a new business course for the medical school and the university far surpasses that of a new building on campus.

It's a value decision between the "show" and the "know."

Free business education sources.

It might be helpful to note here that the Wharton School of Business in the fall of 2013 through the *Coursera* education company sponsorship made available a free course, *An Introduction To Marketing*, presented by Professor of Marketing Barbara E. Kahn, and associates.

> **"Coursera is an education company that partners with the top universities and organizations in the world to offer courses online for anyone to take, *for free*. Our technology enables our partners to teach millions of students rather than hundreds."**
>
> **(From Coursera website)**

The course was presented in such a way that any medical student with no knowledge about marketing could understand and implement easily. But this is just one of many such business learning resources online—*and free at that.*

Amazon.com offers over 250,000 books on the topic of business and marketing. There are numerous *free* and paid business and marketing newsletters as well as blogs that are updated monthly or more frequently.

Unfortunately, medical students are not told about these business resources to learn business principles from. Students would probably not take the time to read them voluntarily, even if they knew all the resources. Their "medical reading" eclipses their "business reading." It's another reason to *require* the business course.

Digital education is moving rapidly to the top of desired methods of education and instruction

Students are so accustomed to DVD, CD, video, and social media communications that they are entertained and learn more quickly with the use of these formats.

Presentation of business courses on all of these digital options could supersede any need for one-on-one lectures. Medical educators know that students today skip lecture classes frequently, which adds to the value of more widespread use of digital learning.

Students vary in their ability to learn depending on the teaching format in which it is presented. Some learn best by reading. Some learn better by hearing (like lectures, podcasts, CDs, and audio). Others learn better by seeing (live lectures, video, DVDs).

This concept about learning is a prominent marketing strategy. The same advertisement or message is presented in multiple formats to connect with more people who will pay attention to the message.

Example of how the business education is received when it's a voluntary program.

The best two ways to effectively encourage use of this communication model is either by providing the whole medical practice business course and training package to each medical student at the beginning of medical school as a free pre-entrance package or to make the package available at a central area where any student has 24/7 access to them.

What would be the predicted cost of providing every medical student in their first year the full business education package? **Would yours be *the first medical school to do that*?**

Most *outside* excellent business-digital-packages promoted by business and marketing experts who teach business courses vary from about $300-$1,500.

The price varies with the amount and type of business materials included. The more expensive packages include such things as DVDs, worksheets, a printed manual that explains everything on the videos. Most also include a bonus DVD on some special aspect of business for free, an introductory DVD to introduce the elements of the package and what information the person will learn with each segment.

Occasionally, the education includes a separate live lecture series on DVD, a live workshop, or a comprehensive live event on the topic with the gurus doing the presentations. The costs of these upgrades commonly cost about $300-$500 for the DVD series, $1,000-$3,000 for workshop registration, and $3,000-$5,000 for live three-day conference event registration.

Travel to and from the event, as well as room rent and food are personal costs that reach about $300 a day and up, depending on the choices of the attendees. Multiplying these average costs by the number of medical students in the class will give a fair estimate of total costs if the business education was outsourced as opposed to in-house.

3. Do the common objections of medical educators stem from legal, economic, or social factors, or from the inertia of an unchangeable belief system bound tightly by their tradition and doctrine thinking about business?

Doctrine = "Telling you what you should believe."

What is least understood about the accountability issue of providing a business education for medical students is the seemingly irrational approach to this issue.

On the one hand, medical education is constantly being updated and adjusted to the newer and most productive medical education nuances that benefit all students (future physicians), and on the other hand education scholars have to be accountable to all medical patients and the national healthcare mandates.

For anyone who understands the full extent of how intricately business knowledge is interwoven with the success, capabilities, and goals of a physician in private practice of medicine, it's difficult to explain why no obvious definitive effort or action has been made by medical schools to seriously consider changing, adapting, or implementing adjunctive solutions.

The egregious nature of such a perpetuation of neglect by the medical educational elite reflects the *true shortsightedness of the medical education system*. It's not unlike sending a soldier into combat with no ammunition for his weapon.

If the stand of the medical education system is to do "just enough" to prepare students for medical practice and nothing more, then the private practice of medicine has been and is now being driven to extinction with the assistance and promotion of the medical education academics.

If the stand of the medical education system has such a narrow focus on teaching medical knowledge and skills only, then their obligation and accountability is in reality not to interpret the common sense "preparation" of students for medical practice as meaning the inclusion of a business education. Such an interpretation is unconscionable.

What accountability really means.

Webster defines **accountable** as, "subject to the obligation to report, explain, or justify something." **Responsible** is defined as, "answerable, accountable as for something within one's power, control, or management—having the capacity for moral decisions—capable of rational thought or actions."

These definitions leave no contrary view about the fact that medical educators are answerable for the ultimate success that every physician has the potential and capacity for. It follows that ultimate success depends on being taught critical business knowledge as much as the medical knowledge. Both are partners in the *complete success* of physicians, medical-wise and business-wise.

About creating accountability where there is none.

If then, the medical education system *lacks a changeable attitude* in regards to providing a formal business education to medical students, *one can conclude that attrition and frustration of physicians will continue and become worse.*

This further implies another detrimental flaw in the minds of academic medical education scholars. Any academic worth his salt should understand that if medical students or doctors disregard the need for a formal business education (and medical school educators already know what it can do for practicing doctors), then someone has to push them, force them, inspire them, persuade them into it by one means or another.

Why? Because it's the right thing to do, starting today.

The negative attitude *about not needing a business education*, documented by the actions of medical students and doctors over the last century, came from somewhere, don't you think? Where would such negative thoughts about never needing a business education come from? God forbid, that the Holy Spirit of God inside them may have gone rogue.

If you think about the possible causes and sources of such beliefs and how they originate, maybe you should also consider the fact that the medical school education system's complete inattention to the necessary business aspect of private medical practice sends an earth-shaking unacceptable message to every medical student.

Obviously, if medical schools *never ever mention the importance of knowing how to run a medical practice business efficiently and profitably*, every medical student gets the subliminal message: that it's not necessary.

Doctors don't ever really seem to "get" the *importance of a business education* to their career. Consequently, they refuse to spend the time to obtain a good business education on their own. I haven't heard a thunderous voice coming down from the clouds in the sky ordering them to comply.

This factor may well spring from the academic's own arrogant attitude, that medical students and physicians already know how "business" works, and they are more than competent to handle that part of medical practice themselves without a formal business education. Such ignorance needs to be rectified.

In essence, medical school educators not only contribute to this belief directly, but also are the manufacturers of doctors who fail to ever reach their maximum career potential: they fail to earn the income they need to reach their original goals and fail to survive in private medical practice. Does the impact that it has on physician *attrition* come to mind?

Is the graduating of physicians who are predestined for failure, a graduate education strategy acceptable to medical school educators? It seems to be the case.

Then the question arises about whether these medical education scholars can be trusted. Logically, if the educators fail to resolve the serious business problems private practice medical doctors have related to the lack of a business education, then where else in the education process are they steering students in the wrong direction?

This skeptical thought can be measured by asking yourself:

a. If only *one medical school* of the one hundred seventy or so medical schools in the USA provided a formal business education along with the normal medical education, would that be the preferred choice of medical school for you to attend?

   One would anticipate that only one of the top twenty medical schools would have the ability and resources to make it happen.

b. If the one medical school offered this double curriculum to medical students, would it solve its recruitment problems, add to its status and prestige among all medical schools, and be in high demand?

It would require that students that apply for entrance need to understand the value of a business education to doctors beforehand to make that decision. This issue should be at the forefront *of "premedical education" dictates.*

c. If this double curriculum was proven to prepare medical students to raise themselves to much higher levels of medical practice skills, knowledge and value to patients, might it widely spread through every medical school in our nation today?

d. Do you believe that it's possible, even probable, that every medical school could create or adopt such a business education program and curriculum for students regardless of the cost, problems, changes, objections, skepticism, and inertia of the educational system to get started?

Might the federal government be interested in subsidizing such a project to improve the healthcare of the nation in this manner?

"When dealing with people, remember you are not dealing with creatures of logic, but with creatures of emotion, creatures bristling with prejudice and motivated by pride and vanity."
-Dale Carnegie

e. Essentially every *successful business owner* agrees that their success requires the continued application and implementation of sound business principles and strategies to maintain that success. Why then is medical practice success and the business of medical practice not subject to the same standards and requirements? **It isn't—at present!**

f. If the introduction of an additional medical school curriculum about business education happened to result in the addition of several months or a year to the medical education process, would it be too much of a financial or time burden to accept? Some medical schools already offer a fifth year to students.

Any doctor with a formal business education is expected to earn twenty times or more than what the cost of the business education was to begin with.

g. If you survey physicians who have been in private medical practice over twenty years and ask them if a formal business education provided at the start of their practice would have benefited them, what would predictably be the predominant response?

Accountability should lead to an actionable progression towards a beneficial goal:

The relationship between accountability and taking action has to be primed by substantiating persuasion. The ears must hear, the eyes must see and the mind must be a willing collaborator for anything to happen.

First, in the business of medical education, medical education scholars must be convinced that the cost, time, effort, and value of providing a business education to medical students will result in more than reasonable benefits to the medical schools as well.

Second, such benefits must also significantly expand the agenda of medical school education far enough to exceed the existing standards and expectations for medical students graduating today. Both the school and students benefit.

Naturally, by agreeing to provide a business education for medical students, the results and benefits must reflect back on the integrity and forward thinking of medical scholars and medical education system in general.

Such a radical yet expeditionary role change in thinking by the medical education elite would surely revolutionize the power and entrepreneurship capabilities of every educational system. The dynamics of all professional businesses would be upgraded across the world. All would adopt them and profit from that decision.

Beyond this view are many more benefits that accompany all well thought-out changes that in the long run will benefit everyone.

4. Why should the medical schools and medical school education system be responsible for providing a business education for medical students in the first place?

Should they do it or not? Presently, they obviously do not want any part of being responsible for additional and especially different educational courses that are seemingly unrelated to teaching students about the practice of medicine.

Who made the rule about medical schools not teaching medical students about the business of medical practice? The private medical practice of medicine can't be sustained without a business foundation. That fact documents the necessity of a business education.

Even though the business of medical practice is an essential foundation for successful private practice of medicine, who decided that a business education of medical students has nothing to do with the process of medical school education and is an unnecessary part of preparing medical students for future medical practice?

Consideration of the assumption that most medical practice educators already know that educating new doctors with both the knowledge and skills of medical practice and the knowledge and skills for business success is the ideal educational objective for graduating the most advanced, valuable, competent, skilled, and productive physicians, then it's simply a matter of how to do it?

In between the ideal objective and the best way to accomplish it are the barriers that can sink the whole project.

The primary barrier is one of making the necessary decisions about the priorities for education of medical doctors.

Would you prefer to have a highly knowledgeable and skilled doctor who is permanently business-compromised in everything he does in private practice throughout his medical career or a doctor who is fully capable of handling both the medical and business sides of his private practice no matter what the threats to practice failure are?

At the same time, medical schools are bent on packing as much medical knowledge into the minds of students as they can, because it mistakenly appears to be a good idea. Educators now equate that process to being a necessity in our world of rapidly increasing changes and improvements in the practice of medicine.

Three questions about "what's enough" medical school education that arise are...

a. What percent of that accumulated medical knowledge is almost never used by doctors later in their medical practice?

Surveys are a simple and credible means of finding out!

Another even more definitive means of checking how much useless information is learned and never used is to survey all the SPEX (exam given by many state boards to candidates for licensure that prior to this exam have been practicing for over ten or fifteen years in another state) licensure exam records and scores.

You may be surprised how many specialty doctors fail the exam because of the huge number of medical details on the test that they have forgotten and have nothing to do with what they have been practicing over the last fifteen years.

b. What are medical schools planning for the inevitable time when medical schools reach a point when the medical information becomes far more than any student can reasonably learn or remember?

Will students be required to attend five or six years of medical school just to learn all the medical information available?

Will students be forced to choose a "specialty" on entrance to medical school, take the curriculum specific for that specialty in two or three years of medical school, and then enter the residency program immediately after that: no internship?

c. Could it be that the addition of a formal medical business education can produce a much more valuable and skilled medical doctor than all those wasted "packed-in" medical education efforts can ever achieve for that doctor?

I submit to you that the true value of providing a formal business education for all medical students is an objective that far outweighs, and should replace, the learned-but-unused medical information being stuffed into the minds of medical students today.

"Whenever you see a successful business, someone once made a courageous decision."
-Peter Drucker

Thoughts that bother an investigative mind:

1. Everyone likely agrees that there is a limit to the amount of medical knowledge that can be learned in a four-year medical school education program. Is the addition of a fifth and sixth year of medical school off the table?

2. Medical scholars and academics may be too close to the medical curriculum requirements to gain a credible and accurate perception of what it takes to enable a medical doctor to perform at his or her highest capabilities. It appears to be so to those of us who are practicing outside of the academic environment.

It seems obvious that every medical student has an imbedded entrepreneurial spirit; otherwise they could not practice medicine with any degree of success.

That willingness to step outside their own knowledge and skills "comfort zone" face medical problems of patients that are often hidden behind unusual symptoms and then stretch their minds to the limit to diagnose and treat the problems makes the medical student and physician unique.

This special characteristic is the ingredient that empowers their ability to handle a formal business education and medical education at the same time. Together, they provide the student a superior foundation for their medical career to grow that is unparalleled in medicine.

In the eyes of intelligent craftsmen and scholars these teaching efforts should be viewed as the creation of a new generation of outstanding physicians that surpass all who have preceded them. Physicians with the capacity to successfully engage the oncoming governmental control and financial restrictions placed on them need the business weapons to fight back. It is an offensive action rather than a defensive one.

Unlike the past generations of doctors who have generally not been able to successfully combat such horrific financial threats because of their total lack of business survival knowledge, they will now have the medical warrior's weapons to use offensively to protect themselves.

Interestingly, I have not encountered during my research any other better *"offensive weapon"* physicians can use to ensure their survival in medical practice than a formal business education.

A physician's sophistication in the knowledge and skills of using business and marketing tools and strategies makes the critical difference in which doctors survive and which won't.

The rising tide of evidence and belief of most business experts today indicate and predict that Obamacare will not be repealed because of the political forces and influences outside of organized medicine.

Assuming that turns out to be the case, any physician without adequate business knowledge will be forced into working for other entities, losing their freedom to practice as they choose, and working as servants (money producers) for the benefit of other entities. It's a heartbreaking thought to even consider.

Sorting out where the responsibility lies.

At present we don't have any volunteers (medical schools, medical scholars, business experts) willing to take on the task of providing a business education for all medical students/doctors. Unfortunately, it has up to today been left up to students and physicians themselves to do it on their own.

Has that approach worked out well in your opinion?

By scanning the number of medical practices failing and the attrition of medical doctors swelling to thousands or more, one has to believe there's a widespread "business virus" killing doctors off in increasing numbers.

Sound reasoning has traced the origin of that viral plague on physicians. The resounding consensus among all who continue to search for ways to save private medical practice is what the elite successful commercial business owners and business experts have been trying to tell us all along.

Without the essential business tools being available and used efficiently, every medical practice in our country has been, and is, predestined to fail from the very start. Practicing doctors routinely reject the advice of business experts or simply don't believe them and resist following advice given to them.

Shamefully, business consultants have had great difficulty getting into a doctor's office, let alone being able to share their business knowledge with doctors one-on-one. Most business experts and consultants have given up trying to penetrate the private medical practice environment; it's not worth the effort. Physicians have driven away an important ally.

There has to be a reason doctors have persistently put up barriers to such essential business knowledge, right?

In light of the opposite reaction (seeking business help) other healthcare providers like dentists, podiatrists, and chiropractors have towards business education, the more bizarre the physician's negative attitude seems to be.

It may be a matter of one of many factors or even a lethal mixture of them. After all, arrogance, fixed mindset, denial and brainwashed beliefs have run through the population of physicians for at least a century.

The defensive nature of physicians concerning the need for business knowledge may be fortified by...

a. Fear about having to learn another whole area of knowledge.

b. The erroneous belief that they can do just as well in their career without formal business knowledge.

c. The belief that the business knowledge will not work for them ("You don't know what you don't know!").

d. Medical schools never emphasized the importance, use, value, and benefits of business knowledge. So the perception about business education by medical students is that it is neither important nor beneficial to physicians.

e. Perhaps, practicing physicians can't afford the time away from their medical practice to obtain the business knowledge, even when they want it and need it.

How many physicians actually voluntarily obtain business education on their own after starting their medical practice? Have you ever been surveyed about that? Very few understand the value of surveys.

Only those who discover the benefits of business knowledge accidentally who have the financial resources to proceed and who are in a position where an MBA will advance their status and opportunities, will benefit. Those medical students who previously obtained an MBA are privileged to be ahead of the game.

Ultimate Fact:
It's not reasonable to expect any graduating medical student to ever obtain a business education on their own.
Reason: They are universally ignorant of the real importance of it to their careers.

To more thoroughly make my point here, a comparison needs to be made. A premedical college student at the point of entering medical school usually has a background accumulation of knowledge only about becoming a doctor.

Often for years, the premedical student has had a compelling focus on and passion for what doctors accomplish, their status in society, the importance of their purpose, and the benefits of being a physician.

They are mentally aware and prepared to obtain the knowledge and skills taught in medical school. They already know the importance and benefits provided by medical education and don't have to be persuaded.

On the other hand, the focus and passion for the *business* of medical practice is non-existent for students entering medical school today as well as throughout their medical school education.

At the time of graduation from medical school, young doctors have no appreciation for, knowledge of, desire built up for, or the drive and passion necessary for top-level business success in medical practice and in their career. Consequently, the importance of obtaining a reliable business education in their minds is relegated to the bottom of the educational totem pole—and they have no reason to go further.

This is why a business education must be provided *during medical school.* Students have to be made aware of and have the time to be persuaded to acknowledge the extraordinary value business education has for all physicians.

Knowing how to manage the business of their future medical practice is not only critical to their eventual success level but also mandatory for their highest accomplishments in medical practice. Most medical students should start with that goal in mind: not a good, but a fantastic physician.

Premedical students know they have to gain the medical knowledge to become a doctor. But they don't know that it also takes a business education to make the most of their personal medical career capabilities—and need to be convinced.

Once they know business knowledge is an essential part of maximal success in medical practice, they predictably will be eager to get it.

Another important factor is the bonding of medical students to the fact that both medical and business education must be recurrently updated for the rest of their medical careers. As medical practice continues to change over time, so does the business of medical practice.

Medical students lead themselves to a medical education, but they must be led, told, and convinced by others about a business education.

This process of adding business education to the curriculums of medical schools is an essential element that can only be accomplished efficiently and productively by medical schools themselves.

Overcoming the resistance of medical education scholars to the addition of business education scheduled during the medical school education process.

First, the process of providing an acceptable business education to students need not, and indeed should not be, provided by the medical school education teaching staff. It belongs to the realm of business experts and the business materials and information they supply. A detailed discussion about this is given in page 132 in chapter 8.

Second, the business curriculum should be *mandatory for students* to participate and should not be provided in any manner that detracts from the medical education curriculum already provided. Yes, it can be done.

Third, it would be appropriate to ask the medical education staff and other associated staff involved in the medical education process to attend the business lecture sessions. Business materials should also be available to the medical staff members—the purpose being that of teaching the medical education staff about the benefits and efficient use of business tools enables them to participate and support the business education staff.

In addition, it enables them to be knowledgeable enough to discuss business strategies with the students when the opportunity presents itself.

The probability that most all of the medical staff themselves have no formal education in business management is common knowledge. How then could they teach it?

"The bonus for the medical teaching staff is that they would be in a position to get a free business education (assuming this has administrative approval) and will benefit from it in many ways themselves. Their value to the school will increase."

Another overlooked advantage provided to physicians is that of using their sound business education to move up to an administrative position within the medical community anywhere, anytime.

If a physician leaves medical practice and starts another career, having a strong business education enables them to find better jobs and rise through the ranks faster than those who don't have a strong business background. This is a win-win situation for all involved.

When all factors are seriously considered, there remains only one determination possible: the addition of a business education curriculum is *the one means of providing a "complete" medical career education for all physicians.* It's something that pride in such an unbelievable accomplishment falls short of describing the fulfillment one enjoys well enough.

There is no debate about the fact that all people engaged in this mission are accountable and responsible in their own way for business education becoming a major pillar and standard for a dedicated medical school education platform at a much higher level.

Skepticism plays a positive part in adding a business education to the medical education system.

Who says that a business education does anything to benefit any physician practicing medicine? It would take a mental IQ of 60 to believe there is no benefit, even if it involved learning only the simple means of getting along well with others, such as your patients.

For physicians who either take administrative positions or quit medical practice completely, a keen knowledge of business increases the probability of transitioning to another job or career with ease. Physicians with this knowledge become an asset for patients, hospitals, and the healthcare system regardless of their purpose in life or the status they hold. It's a formidable asset to their children and family as well.

Individuals who spout negative slams about business education of medical students are those who can't be helped unless somehow they become enlightened about business principles, acknowledge the benefits, and have experience to substantiate that business education makes a significant difference. Skepticism can be erased by learning the truth.

"The characteristic that tends to distinguish the winners from the losers is the relentless conversion of problems to opportunities, negatives to positives."
-Dan S. Kennedy

Skepticism, when rebutted by overwhelming evidence to the contrary, stimulates the open-minded person to investigate why their position is threatened. In doing so, they come to realize that the truth is often camouflaged by the lack of education about the issue.

Continued skepticism is the prime trigger for failure because action is never taken to resolve the issue or to discover the truth.

Everyone has some skepticism about something. The cure is always more knowledge. Skepticism is erased and converted into decisions.

Elsewhere, I mentioned the fact that business consultants have given up on trying to educate physicians about the beneficial aspects of business knowledge. Physicians who have no formal business knowledge will ensure that this dilemma will persist forever.

A converted skeptic is the best promoter of the issue at hand. I relate to that person in a highly emotional way because I'm a converted skeptic regarding the value of a business education of physicians and is why I write this book today.

"Success means doing the best we can with what we have. Success is the doing, not the getting; in the trying, not the triumph. Success is a personal standard, reaching for the highest that's in us, becoming all that we can be."
-Zig Ziglar

CHAPTER 5

The Triage

"Career-Long Decisive Benefits are Created for All Physicians When They are Armed with a Formal Business Education that Benefits Everyone"

The business of medical practice becomes a formidable ally for the optimal success of medical practice only when a new doctor has been taught the parameters and discipline of using proven and trusted business success tools.

MEDICAL PRACTICE IS, and always has been, understood to be a significant small business entity. For any physician to be the most efficient and productive in medical practice, they must have a formal business education.

That's not debatable among those academics that stand for a "**complete**" education of medical students preparing for a long life of practicing medicine.

At present, medical students are being *prepared only for half of the private practice of medicine*: that of actual care and treatment of human illness and trauma. Business ignorance limits all doctors' ability to do so.

The other half of the private practice of medicine is learning how to create, manage, and perpetuate the business of medical practice, something that has never been provided over the last century.

When any physician lacks significant formal business education, they are being deprived of major business elements required for maximal success in their profession and medical practice.

It's gambling with a doctor's future when their professional career is being left to circumstances and fate. When a medical practice reaches the edge of financial failure, it's unsustainable and has no options for survival.

That's a gamble our everyday private practice physicians currently face: without having the backup business knowledge of a formal business education to reverse the process. A formal business education goes even further.

Business education enables any doctor to recognize the signs of financial failure in their practice early enough to use the business tools to prevent it from happening. This financial trap is becoming a common occurrence in private practice today *all because of a lack of business knowledge* among physicians.

It is equally important to drive your *medical practice business* to its maximal potential as it is to expand the capabilities of your medical practice beyond the limits you originally believed you were capable of accomplishing.

Both medical practice and medical practice business, working in tandem, provide physicians with the ultimate use of their knowledge and skills for the benefit of their patients and for the documentation of the integrity and essence of the medical profession.

The compelling effects of self-imposed limitations.

Self-limitations that doctors commonly place on themselves, their capabilities and their optimal performance, are the most influential factors that subconsciously inhibit the ability of doctors to elevate themselves above the usual mediocrity of medical practice performance and profitability.

Anyone who has read "Gerber's *The E-myth: Physician*" has a clear understanding of why so often the great majority of physicians fail to reach their peak in their medical practice careers and why they reluctantly settle for being satisfied with "good enough" in their practice growth, efficiency, and productivity.

The dishonor that the perpetuation of this "mediocrity" blindfold places on the whole medical profession is real, but it can be rectified quite easily and promptly if you know how and take action.

Without a doubt, the only choice of accepting a "mediocre" medical practice to nurture along for years is a direct result of having no reliable business knowledge of how to change their financial situation physicians are encumbered with. Physicians are left to accept what circumstances have dictated to them when they have no clue about business alternatives that can rescue them over and over again.

Doctors don't need more medical education nor do they need to work harder by seeing more patients every day. What they do need at that time in their careers is a boatload of essential business knowledge.

Almost all doctors lack formal business education. They are never told that it's necessary. They are never offered, let alone provided, with business education during their medical education training.

Once they graduate, they are mentally compelled to avoid stopping their medical practice long enough to obtain the business education they need. When their medical career gets down to the level of survival, human behavior will always grasp for money rather than for a business education and more debt.

Losing time and the loss of income from their medical practice to obtain business education happens at exactly the worst time in their careers, when educational debt needs to be paid back, they have no other job or source of income, and it's difficult to get another loan, if not impossible.

Every graduating medical student knows what may well be required of them: to become an employee. The rapidly increasing trend today among graduating medical students is to get a "medical practice job" and earn money on a salary. In this position they become the sacrificial lamb of the employer and earn money for the employer instead of themselves.

It's sad but true.

"If you have a poor financial education,
you will always work for the rich."
-Robert Kiyosaki

Providing a formal business education for all medical students is the *most effective solution* to the attrition of physicians troubling our present-day healthcare system!

The *business* education of medical students is a unique and an extraordinary benefit to every counterpart of medical education.

1. **Benefits to medical schools.**

    a. Medical schools that understand the marketing value of this medical education undertaking will dominate the respect and admiration of all other medical schools while maximizing the school's reputation and desirability.

    b. Medical schools that implement the business education of students and who graduate doctors that are armed with business knowledge and tools streamlined for higher levels of medical practice business success have an unprecedented opportunity to lead the practice of medicine from the top.

    c. The recognition of a higher demand for business integration into medical student curriculums in an economic environment of increasingly controlled and restricted medical fees and physician incomes needs compensatory action.

    The action taken indicates the outstanding commitment of medical scholars to ensure the *complete* preparedness of medical doctors to practice medicine at much higher achievable levels of success in adapting appropriately to increased economic restrictions in the future.

    If only one medical school is doing this, the benefits to that medical school are multiplied exponentially. When more medical schools implement a similar business education system, the marketing benefits are diluted.

    d. The first to implement the business education breakthrough in medical school education always receives the most response, publicity, and media attention especially when it is a revolutionary advancement in medical education. The first to do it will always maintain the top threshold of educational advancement and be remembered for that incredible display of educational integrity to be the best.

e. Benefits extend to increased gifts and donations from the medical school alumni who earn more, appreciate their education more, and pay back more. Other equally important benefits to medical schools can be found in the public relations, marketing, promotional, referral and recommendations, ratings, recruiting, and administration areas.

f. Medical schools benefit much more when their medical students are capable of continued advancements in medical practice far above those who don't know business. Any graduate that becomes well known for their expertise, leadership, and prestige reflects back on the medical school where they were trained.

2. The benefits and institutional rewards for teaching business principles to medical students.

The continuous flow of mail from the alumni groups and medical institutions to all physicians never ends. Soliciting donations from former graduates is even more critical and necessary today because of the government cutting back on financial support to hospitals and medical schools to avoid total collapse of our economy.

It's reasonable to assume that physician's donations are used for medical student scholarships and the financial needs of the medical schools. It implies that medical schools are not able to stand on their own revenue production.

The alternative would be to raise the tuition so high that applicants to the school would find it totally unaffordable except to a rare few, but it would cover the schools expenses and not require financial donors to cover the medical education process. It's not a good idea.

Now think, what would happen if every graduate was equipped with a formal business education from the start of their medical practice? Certainly the physician donations back to their schools would be expectedly elevated to levels that would make history. Is it unrealistic to think so?

My experience and incomplete knowledge about the statistics concerning doctors who donate back to schools and those who don't, as well as the amounts donated by the various categories of those doctors, leaves me only the choice of guessing what those statistics reveal regarding each medical school.

It would not surprise me that *75 percent of every medical school class* never donates anything back to their school during their medical careers. Furthermore, if medical schools and universities are able to persuade even 5 percent of their alumni to donate more than $1,000 during their whole medical careers, it would surprise me. What would you believe the reason could be for such low contributions by so many alumni?

Of course, those statistics are closely held by all schools and rarely available to all alumni. On rare occasions, I see a classmate of mine who has donated to the school in our medical school alumni magazine.

The strategy often used to draw donors is to publish a targeted list of those who donated an amount that put their name on the bronze, silver, gold, or platinum levels or categories (a very productive marketing method appealing to the personal recognition, pride, status, and other emotional elements of the donor).

The belief that donations from alumni would increase significantly if physicians were able to earn much more in their medical practices, seems logical. It follows that because of having an extensive knowledge of business and the business tools required, much higher donations would occur proportionally.

One then must pose the question as to why this strategy is apparently not supported by all medical schools because of this potential income benefit.

Good results from this kind of soliciting have been reported. The May 5, 2014 edition of *Forbes* magazine reported Princeton's alumni private donations reached a median of $29,330 and alum participation rate of 46 percent. The study related to a ten-year span divided by the number of undergrad students. It impressed me even if it wasn't a medical school survey (See www.forbes.com/gratefulgrads). It documents that return on investment is linked to the quality of graduates they produce.

The additional benefits of graduating medical doctors who are all educationally equipped business-wise to far exceed the status, accomplishments, and leadership that other medical school's graduates will never attain. It offers the opportunity for a school to expand on their reputation, desirability, and prominence in the medical educational system hierarchy.

Doing *what other medical schools are not doing* for their medical students is a foundational principle of marketing that is above reproach. Any academic institution that institutes a revolutionary change and benchmark is in a unique position to receive benefits that happen only once in a lifetime.

The effect of such a celebration is a rare public relations breakthrough for any medical education accomplishment. Such achievements, as rare as they are, are associated with such an institution indefinitely. Who would not want to have it mentioned in medical profession education history books that your medical school is on the cutting edge in the field?

3. Benefits to physicians.

a. Physicians know that after they graduate from medical school that provided them an additional business education, they are *far more confident in their ability to meet the challenges* created by changes in the economy, the medical profession, and their personal financial status if need be. Opportunities increase.

b. With a sound business education, all graduating medical students are armed with the business tools that will prevent them from having to confront medical practice business financial failure, loss of practice income from medical practice competition, and loss of patients from referral doctors, among others.

c. Business knowledge enables new physicians to set up their medical practice at a place and in the right circumstances that are known to enable practice business growth and income. Otherwise, it's guesswork or hope that where they decided to start practice will meet their needs.

d. Physicians with a formal business education can grow their practice multiple times faster, expand their practice persistently, and recognize the signs of financial failure early enough to correct the problems.

e. Physicians who have a good business education are much better doctors than they would have been otherwise because they understand that the more income they have the more medical education and skills they have access to and can afford. They already have the business tools to conveniently increase their income as often as needed for business or personal gain.

f. Physicians with essential formal business knowledge position themselves to be in high demand by recruiters, medical partnerships, organized medicine, medical school teaching staff, and administrative medicine positions, among others.

g. If business-educated physicians should be forced to leave medical practice for some compelling reason, they are already prepared and qualified for many more job opportunities in business outside of medicine. In our present state of increasing physician attrition, business education becomes far more important to doctors.

4. **Benefits to employed physicians and their employers.**

Regardless of where, how, or when a physician becomes endowed with a formal business education, such a physician becomes a formidable asset to their own or any other organization they work with or under.

The exciting part of being a business-educated professional is that their knowledge, competency, management skills, and business capabilities added to their core medical education makes them a rare professional in high demand in any workplace.

These outstanding educational attributes together not only widens their professional capabilities in the medical job market, but also paves the way to a much higher level of accomplishments. Such a physician becomes considerably more valuable to any medical business entity, whether it is a hospital, HMO, medical education, research, or other related medical business.

For one thing, this dual capability and knowledge eliminates the need for two employees: one does it all. Looking at trends presently visible in healthcare, wouldn't the increasing need for physician administrators be obvious? Wouldn't any hospital board prefer a CEO with both qualifications?

The likelihood of far increased salary benefits resulting from this dual education certainly would exceed those expected from most private medical practice businesses.

Undoubtedly, any physician who finds it necessary for one of many reasons to leave the practice of medicine could easily transition into an administrative position inside or outside the medical profession.

Certainly, competition with the American College of Physician Executives and the American College of Healthcare Executives would have to be negotiated or allied with the medical school curriculum to some extent.

Other more practical benefits sprout from these roots as well. What do you think would happen when one medical school suddenly started graduating all medical students with this dual capability? Rightly, that school would quickly become the choice for recruitment of their graduates by every employer in the nation having the need for such professionals.

Think about the escalating benefits that would then become available to that medical school, other than being the dominant medical school for educating physicians. That exceptional reputation would pull the eyes and ears of the world to its front steps.

Some quick calculations might tell you that such a medical school would draw the attention of philanthropic organizations who know the necessity and value of such a futuristic educational venture, and be more than willing to justify it with their contributions to it.

5. **Benefits for medical students.**

a. There is no more fertile time to grasp the essential and successful business principles, including marketing, than while medical students are undergoing medical education and at the most inspired time in their medical career to accept a second educational process that is tightly bound to their success in medical practice.

b. When students are molding their future careers in medicine, the application of business knowledge permits them to apply the aspects of business education to their career decision making at the same time. The two educational processes (medical and business) working together enable students not only to make more satisfactory decisions about their career, but also the key to making decisions that are more in line with their personal motivations and goals.

c. Learning about business while in medical school enables students to clearly recognize the value and importance of how medical practice business serves to complement their career, not inhibit it. In a true sense it plants the urgency for a lifelong thirst for continued business education along with the thirst for ongoing medical education.

d. For students who have essentially no business education or background experience in business, the integration of business knowledge into their medical education is much more effective and advantageous than later realizing the need for and importance of business knowledge. That's when formidable barriers present themselves and deter any inspiration to obtain a business education.

e. A student's mind is highly primed for learning during their medical education. It is primed by motivation when they are in an inspirational environment as well as builds their desire and passion to learn much more than what most scholars associate with a medical students capabilities at the time.

It's the entrepreneurial attitude implanted in the minds of all medical students to go beyond what they expect from themselves—and they do it over and over with the help of mentoring.

Personally, I never believed that I was capable of learning the origin and insertions of every muscle in the human body, but I did it.

f. The reasons that a formal business education for medical students has to be provided during their medical school education process is because that education will only sink in if a student is put into direct contact with the medical professionals and can experience the practice business issues first hand and with a mentor.

It's no different than really learning medicine by immersing students in real patients with real medical problems. When a student learns it all from books, DVDs, and other digital formats, it won't be remembered as well nor be as conveniently applicable to their own future in medicine. Business becomes important and remembered through real experience.

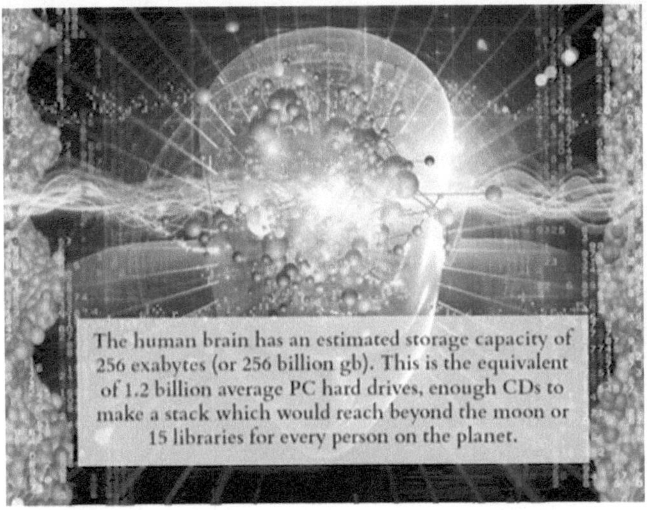
The human brain has an estimated storage capacity of 256 exabytes (or 256 billion gb). This is the equivalent of 1.2 billion average PC hard drives, enough CDs to make a stack which would reach beyond the moon or 15 libraries for every person on the planet.

6. Benefits to our society and medical patients

a. The ability to become a much more qualified physician by knowing how to manipulate their medical practice business income using business principles results in the ability to afford any and all training they choose. With adequate income there is no limitation to advancement.

When equipped with more polished skills, training, and knowledge, they become the center of attraction of patients, referrals, and consultations as a result of the continued improvement of their skills. It makes every physician in that scenario a better doctor in all ways and for all patients.

b. With the accumulation of more skills and medical knowledge, physicians are able to offer patients more services, treatments, and options for care rather than having to refer patients to other doctors for care that already have the skills.

   Medical patients much prefer that their own doctor do as much as possible for their healthcare rather than be referred out. It's also a prime means for improvement of the doctor-patient relationship as well.

c. Consider a hundred or a thousand physicians with a formal business education under their belt, able to do all that's described above for their patients. The idea has to be held as one of the most fantastic improvements in healthcare across all medical specialties and the medical profession—if such a business education is provided.

7. **Future benefits to healthcare in the USA.**

Medical technology is rapidly improving medical care by doctors and predictably will continue to escalate. However, the probability of the continued deterioration of private medical practice and the independence of doctor's healthcare decision-making will not be cured by new digital medical technology.

However, by combining a formal business education of medical students with the advancing medical technology, the advancement in medical care and all healthcare will most certainly skyrocket in quality.

That leap will occur because the platform on which all medical practice functions most effectively is based on a business structure. Just try practicing medicine without any business platform sometime. Think like a cash-only practice in a cardboard hut on a corner in downtown NYC.

Physicians who know how to manage a successful business will always remain at the top of their medical practice game.

Just imagine what healthcare would be like if every graduating new doctor had a firm grip of business knowledge from the start of their practice, regardless of where and how they choose to practice. The full extent of this one change and improvement of healthcare can't be predicted, but would certainly be overwhelming in dimension.

Samuel Huntington, author of the book entitled, *"The Third Wave,"* seemed to have a futuristic grasp of the lessons in history that the new generation disregards: *"The West (our nation) that consistently sacrifices efficiency on the altars of regulation, litigation and political consensus will lose the dynamism that makes the risks inherent in free societies seem worthwhile."*

It can quite appropriately be applied to the regulation, litigation, and political consensus concerning the medical profession and the attrition of physicians today. The same causes create the same results. (Quoted by Bret Stephens in *WSJ* April 22, 2014).

CHAPTER 6

The Wound Cause

"Universal Business Principles, when Understood and Implemented are Key to the Maximum Success of Any Business, Including Medical Practice"

If the ultimate purpose of any medical practice business is for it to reach the level of productivity and profitability that enables the accomplishment of every goal of the physician owner, then the knowledge, application, and implementation of business principles are absolutely required.

For any inspired physician who desires to reach their personal optimal potential and capabilities in their private medical practice career, nothing short of an academic business education will assure that it happens.

THE ESTABLISHED AND foundational business principles for any business's success are the same and never change. The application and effectiveness of those principles do change frequently over time depending on what is required to maintain persistent growth, profitability, and end game.

Understanding how to apply those business principles and strategies to any doctor's medical practice business is the obligation of every physician who desires to maximize their value to their patients and the medical profession.

A formal business and marketing education is required for physicians who have a passion for reaching their peak potential. Otherwise, physicians who aren't provided with that education are predestined to continue with a medical career of continued financial thirst with no economic watering hole in sight.

The deluge of bad consequences resulting from the lack of a business education is seen every day across the medical profession. The worst consequence of all is that physicians are led to believe that a formal business education is not necessary (at least no one told them about its value) for an optimal successful medical practice.

And there begins the difficult task of defining what medical practice success means. Understandably, every physician defines success in a different manner, depending on their own goals, motivation level, and what they believe is the limit of their ability to do any better.

About 97 percent of physicians enter private practice with little or no idea of what they are capable of in their medical career. Self-ascribed limitations, unrealistic goals, lack of planning, lack of due diligence, variable amounts of determination, and inertia are some of the troublesome issues that result in scattering of energy and efforts on multiple tasks and loss of self-esteem and self-confidence.

These are the things that lead to failure in medical practice, mediocrity in medical practice, and accepting everything measured by the criteria of "good enough" to get by.

Most all of these career influencing problems are resolved when the entrepreneurial spirit is invigorated by having a clear view of how success works—and that few doctors seem to recognize in themselves.

The knowledge acquired from a formidable business education can and does reverse the majority of problems physicians have today, both inside and outside of the business of medical practice.

The satisfaction resulting from this basic security is what pulls doctors out of "fear and worry" and into "confidence and new ambition." It's fostered by an understanding that good business foundations are what enable a medical practice to succeed. The extent and quality of the *business foundation* for medical practice then determines the height of success and productivity.

For employed physicians, success is not defined by themselves.

Employed physicians are provided security backed by the employer or organization that hired them. Their business foundation is already provided and in place with risk of failure being spread across the full business system components.

Employed physicians are separated from those who run the business side of the company and therefore the passion of and desirability for success is measured by and limited to the success defined by the organization, not by the individual physician.

Employed physicians never have to understand how success works because even that is out of their own control. For doctors that are employees there is no necessity for a business education or responsibility for obtaining it. But, there are many other good reasons for doing it.

However, it's totally different for the small (surveys show about 15 percent) number of physicians who leave medical employers and start a private medical practice.

Remember, nearly all physicians who have sold their medical practice, quit practice, or have lost their practice for one reason or another find that the cause of their action is nearly always a deficiency of adequate practice income.

"Hardly anything in life can be accomplished without money."
-Anonymous

The true nature of success falls far short of entrepreneurism and ultimate business profitability.

Most physicians in private practice define financial success by their reaching a balance between what they can earn in practice and the satisfaction they get from that income. If they find a way to earn more, then their satisfaction with medical practice goes up and their lifestyle improves.

That's the reason working harder, working longer hours, and seeing more than the usual number of patients daily is mistakenly believed to be the best way to elevate income and satisfaction. Working harder is not the answer because there are physical, emotional, and stress factors that become intolerable over a short period of time.

Working smarter is the answer.

How do you do that? It's the question nearly all physicians confront sooner or later in their private practice. Most physicians have no idea how to work smarter because they haven't been told how. Consequently, they simply stop the struggle and accept what the circumstances offer them.

This reactive response to circumstances is the greatest tragedy of private medical practice today. Thousands upon thousands of doctors spend their medical careers accomplishing only a smidgen of what they are capable of doing without realizing that there is a way to pull themselves out of the financial and emotional quicksand.

The secret that explains how to work smarter is what has been intentionally hidden from all medical doctors for a couple centuries. It's something that medical education scholars take no responsibility for and something that even the mention of bristles the hair on the back of the neck of all medical education academics.

It's something that all successful commercial business owners have known for eons and laugh at the physicians about. That "permissive disconnect" from business education is an important primary cause of failure in the business of medical practice.

Physicians and other professional healthcare providers are deeply wounded by not being told the real truth about business success requirements early enough to make a difference in the careers of every doctor.

The whole purpose of a *business education* is to teach anyone how to start a business, manage a business successfully, and how to effectively use business tools to work smarter instead of harder. Business tools do that while providing solutions to all the issues that cause doctors to fail in their medical practice businesses.

Every physician who understands this should be furious about this *unexplained enigma* in the medical profession hierarchy today.

Academics who have neglected this responsibility should be ashamed for ignoring this critical element in a medical student's education.

In a sense, medical students over the years have been being quietly prepared for becoming "employed" physicians only, where business knowledge is not required. Has that been the secret objective and agenda of organized medicine all these years?

The fact is, the business of medical practice, as every successful medical business owner does know without question, requires a *business-educated physician* to run the business efficiently and profitably at peak rate during their whole medical career.

When that business education happens, physicians have no significant barriers to unlimited income, practice growth, improvements of medical skills, medical education, and opportunities for advancement in professional status and value to our nation's health management.

The critical impact factor that can change the lives and practices of thousands of doctors for the better.

The instinctual behavior of doctors who don't know how to go about improving their medical practice business is to give up and settle for the "ordinary" practice life of inertia. However, their entrepreneurial spirit begs to be released every day through all those years of education and medical practice challenges.

Every physician can recognize through introspection that they have that entrepreneurial gift, but don't know what it takes to open up the process and use it. The trigger that releases that spirit in physicians is another educational gift—business knowledge.

**"Never mistake knowledge for wisdom.
One helps you make a living; the other
helps you to make a life."**
-Sandra Carey

That single event when it happens makes an incredible change not only in the fact that they have acquired an amazing aptitude for problem solving that goes beyond comprehension, but also have suddenly acquired the ability to extend their objectives far beyond their expectations without the fear of failure.

Entrepreneurship surfaces when one recognizes what things have been holding them back. Usually those things are the erroneous mental beliefs that have been implanted in their minds since birth.

Belief that the brain is limited in its capacity to store information and then to extract that information for use from our memory banks to be used later, is a common one, but is not true.

More practical factors that hinder our progress include self-ascribed limitations, lack of due diligence, lack of understanding that failure is nothing more than a reason to try another path, the numerous fears and doubts about our own abilities, and lack of recognition that you don't know what you don't know.

All of the above well-known factors are some of the ways one can describe an entrepreneurial spirit.

> **The usual definition of an entrepreneur:** *"Someone who understands that there are solutions to every problem, that stepping out of their comfort zone opens the subconscious mind to perform marvelous insight and supportive information that under usual circumstances is unavailable, and that the process of one's thinking from that point on is purely amazing and continuous."*

The process and the manner in which it happens can be found in *Psycho-Cybernetics*, a book written by Maxwell Maltz, MD, plastic surgeon, (1899-1975) about 1960 and updated in 2001. The book has changed the lives of well over thirty million people and the information has remained unchallenged to the present day.

The book should be required reading for every medical student who has any desire to be the best that they can be.

"If we did all the things in life
we are capable of doing we would
literally astound ourselves."
-Thomas Edison

The use of "business systems" is key to the optimal productivity of any private medical practice and key to the retention, satisfaction, and fulfillment of all physicians.

By any standard of business success, the implementation of *business systems* into any medical practice office will magnify every element of medical practice that has to do with increasing income, profits, and ultimate success of the practice and owner.

Healthcare professionals, from doctors to physical therapists, who have their own businesses, often look for help in the wrong places. They go through their careers constantly battling the outside forces that incessantly try to control their businesses.

Almost all medical practice business owners lose money every day because of their ignorance about what a business system is or that they even exist. Business systems are the series of engines that add to the bottom lines of businesses.

The products created by business systems are productivity, efficiency, and profitability.

Businesses that never use any form of business systems are guaranteed to fail. The same result occurs in medical practice offices as well. What most physicians don't recognize is that they are already using simple, unnoticed forms of business systems in their private practices.

There's always a reason. Doctors either weren't taught, were never educated in business principles, or never understood that *there is a permanent cure for profitless businesses.*

Medical practice businesses tend not to survive when they are subject to a business foundation based on a learn-as-you-go creation process.

You'll discover that all the remarkably effective marketing strategies presently used in the world of business never solve your problems alone with creating a sustainable profitable business.

It's only then that your attention is drawn to the necessity of having an organized business structure and foundation that will enable marketing efforts to create the results they are designed to accomplish.

Business Systems + Marketing = Profits

Successful and profitable medical businesses require *both* a business system infrastructure and marketing strategies that bring in new medical patients to your medical practice on a regular continuing basis.

Successful business is composed of a series of coordinated, synergized, and compatible systems working in unison towards a specific objective.

A Sample Business System Overview.

The definition of a business system for a medical business is defined as a *dynamic balance of the six major foundational components of your business*:

- **Financial Logistics**
- **Internal Processes**
- **Innovation**
- **Learning**
- **Growth**
- **Patient Management**

My articles on my medical website related to this issue are: www.MarketingAMedicalPractice.com

- Article_20.htm
- Article_21.htm
- Article_18.htm
- Article_G.htm

The supreme business guru known throughout the world as the *father of business management*, *Peter Drucker*, whose books about business management continue to be read and used almost a century later, says it all:

A business has only two functions: *marketing and innovation.*

He meant that the functional components of any business have these two objectives. In the process of reaching these objectives, it's necessary to create business systems and processes that support those objectives. What spins off from that effort is what we superficially know as business revenue, profitability, productiveness, and business stability/growth.

Detailed line by line descriptions of personal office business systems should be written down and kept in a three-ring binder. Anyone in your medical business office then has immediate access to the pages of information defining in detail how your office will function under most all circumstances. Don't you think that this sounds incredibly like having an *Employee Policy and Procedures Manual*? You bet.

Chris Anderson's business (www.*BizManualz.com*) of providing you with various business manuals, starter information, and a newsletter with excellent information articles, is one of the best resources on the topic.

Business systems need to be created, or at least modified from a template, to mesh with the ultimate objective that the business owner has established, because the system will be unique to each medical practice setup.

No one else has the same ideas, desires, goals, and plans for their business system as you do. Does it take time and concentration to create the system? Absolutely. Anything worthwhile requires work and time to implement.

The good part is that once it's completed, any revisions later are done in a matter of minutes over the next forty years in practice. Judging from the present trends in the medical profession, most physicians and other doctors may not be in private practice in fifteen to twenty years, if that.

Business System Components

First, you define the ultimate goal or mission for your medical practice. For example, is your aim to make money fast and retire early?

Or is it your desire to have a medical practice that is stable and provides the income necessary to live a simple life? It's any goal you choose for your career and profession.

Once that is determined, a business system compatible with creating that goal can be created.

The critical aspect is to ensure that every element of that system is pulling in the same direction. The elements of the business system dealing with employees have to accomplish the integration of their efforts with a focus on the ultimate growth and expansion to meet the objectives of your business.

Alignment and compatibility of every aspect of the various components has to be clearly planned out. Breaking the business system down to its roots is the next step.

In a simplified way, it looks like this:

Business System → Business Functions → Each Business Function → Business Processes → Process Mapping → Education.

Business System—
-sequential system of goals established
-reasons for creating the systems
-understanding the system's value to the medical business

Business Functions (some)
-accounting, bookkeeping, records
-management, levels and accountability
-patient acquisition and recruitment methods
-supplies and inventory resources and backup
-planning and administration functions
-marketing strategies, including plans
-growth goals and timing, and opportunity
-competition factors and solutions
-continued business education and updates
-communications and interactions required

Individual Business Functions—
-list of processes needed to perform that function
-list of projects that each function can perform
-establish and record compatible interactions among processes
-ways to improve the system processes
-ways to save time and effort

Business Processes (how you actually do the job)
-take each process and break it down into steps
-list of steps in the order of performance
-define the value (contribution) of each step
-how to make each step more efficient
-use of deadlines for work efforts

Process Mapping (mind impact is greater with)
-diagrams, flowcharts, graphs, images
-value it provides for learning and efficiency
-simplifies any complex system by presentation models

Education
-teaching every employee the business system steps
-refreshing sessions so they don't forget
-employee cooperation is dependent on reminders and oversight
-a system is useless without everyone participating in a coordinated fashion

This simplified outline should be a guide *for creating a medical business system*. It means doctors must dig down into the areas of their practice business that they detest doing and have no desire to even think about.

A *much higher level of business profitability and success* is the reward for going the extra mile to set it up. This exercise forces doctors to learn every aspect of how their business functions and what each process accomplishes.

Less than one doctor in thirty thousand ever gets to this level of knowledge about his medical practice business, which is probably why so many medical practice businesses fail.

Paying to have this project done can be expensive, but there usually are fill-in-the-blanks templates for business systems available online to use.

To win, doctors must be smart business people, especially in our medical practice environment of decreasing incomes, failing economic system, and failing political system. The battle up to now has been "*defensively fought*" by all entities supporting our profession. We can now go on the "*offense*" because of what I am proposing be implemented.

Template for a medical marketing plan

Below is an example of a marketing plan, proven and tempered, that escapes the dogma proliferated from the halls of education and defines itself from the battleground experiences of the work ethic:

"Getting the right message to the right people via the right media and methods… effectively, efficiently, and profitably."
---Dan S. Kennedy

The profile of this business expert is shown below.

Dan S. Kennedy is a serial multi-millionaire entrepreneur, a highly paid and sought after marketing and business strategist, an advisor to countless first-generation from-scratch multi-millionaire and seven-figure income entrepreneurs and professionals and, in his personal practice, one of the very highest-paid direct-response copywriters in America. As a speaker, he has delivered over two thousand compensated presentations, appearing repeatedly on programs with the likes of Donald Trump, Gene Simmons (KISS), Debbi Fields (Mrs. Fields Cookies), and many other celebrity-entrepreneurs, for former U.S. presidents and other world leaders, and other leading business speakers like Zig Ziglar, Brian Tracy, and Tom Hopkins, often addressing audiences of one thousand to ten thousand and up. His popular books have been favorably recognized by *Forbes, Business Week, Inc.*, and *Entrepreneur.* His *NO B.S. MARKETING LETTER*, one of the business newsletters published for members of GKIC Insider's Circle, is the largest paid subscription newsletter in its genre in the world.

Create your own marketing plan:

Mr. Kennedy's approach to a marketing plan is a brilliant series of questions that serve to bypass the confusion that ordinary definitions and interpretations often create. Read the following five questions that will provide a starting place for anyone in any business, *especially the business of medical practice.*

1. **Is your marketing built around the most powerful, persuasive, intriguing, compelling, fascinating message possible?**

   (Or is your message ordinary, me-too-ish, dull, mundane, unexciting, plain vanilla, just-the–facts-ma'am, easily ignored, very forgettable? Or, worse, just about a commodity? Or worse still, just about cheap or lowest price?)

2. **Have you determined precisely who your message should be for and figured out how to put it in front of them, quite possibly at the exclusion of all others or at least with disregard for all others?**

   (Or are you a vague generality, for anybody—and thus for nobody? Are you dissipating rather than concentrating your marketing firepower, trying to be noticed and heard by a population far greater in size than your resources?)

3. **Are you wisely investing in the most appropriate media for delivery of your message to the prospects in your chosen target market?**

(Or are you using media because everybody else seems to be, or it is popular or has a salesperson arrived and pushed you into it, or because it's the way you've always operated?
Note: Different media are best for different businesses and different target markets at different times.)

4. **Are you both effective and efficient?**

   (Or are you choosing the easiest, the simplest, or the most efficient means out of laziness or ignorance or "too busyness" or in surrender to recalcitrant employees or poverty consciousness and cheapskate behavior?)

5. **Are you accurately measuring the true, net return on investment from each marketing investment?**

   (Or not? Or guessing? Or carrying around opinions not verified by fact?)

This information is taken directly from Dan Kennedy's book, "*The Ultimate Marketing Plan*" Fourth Edition 2011. It is undoubtedly the most realistic and understandable book on the topic in the world today.

The general understanding about what marketing is makes it much simpler to understand.

Marketing is *what you do* from the time an idea, service, or product comes to mind, until the service (medical practice) is sold to a buyer, feedback is obtained, and the buyer is satisfied.

"What you do" means that you create something that is in demand and then do everything that's necessary to sell the product to the right buyer at the right time, at the right price, and repeat that process over and over. This is exactly what every physician does every day in medical practice.

For physicians it means you started with the passion to be a doctor, then acquired the education you needed. After that, you sell the services you are now an expert in to the patients who need it. There are many other factors that can either interfere with your progress or magnify your progress. Those you learn from a formal business education along with a medical education.

You are welcome to download and read my eBook, at no cost. The URL address is in the caption of the book cover graphic.

"The Business of Medical Practice"

Please Note: A copy of this iconic eBook is available to you on my website.

"A formal education will make you a living,
Self-education will make you a fortune."
-Jim Rohn

CHAPTER 7

Business System Basics

"Effective and Profitable Businesses are Not Characterized by Their Benefits, but by the Creation of 'Business Systems' that Enable the Perpetuation of the Benefits for as Long As Needed"

The ultimate objective of a business system is to provide a repeatable and easily adaptable method for increasing the profitability and efficiency of a business without having to compromise any aspect of the work force efforts in doing so.

PHYSICIANS ARE RESPONSIBLE for the creation of their own *business system* for their own medical practice. No one else has the foggiest idea of what a doctor's personal objectives are for their own medical practice business.

The physician usually has goals in mind for the practice and knows how he or she prefers that they be accomplished. Hiring an expert to do it leads to confusion, wrong interpretations, and the eventual dissatisfaction of the physician employer.

It occurs because no amount of discussion between the hired consulting expert and physician about the project will prevent the biases and "superior" knowledge of the expert from being introduced into or in place of the physician's instructions and ideas.

The other problem is that changes will always have to be made later and who better to make those than the doctor-owner? Maybe the doctor wants to see more patients each day? Maybe he needs to update his doctor referral system as new doctors come into town and wants to increase his number of doctor-referred patients to his/her own practice?

The fact that over 60 percent of new patients in any medical practice are the result of *doctor referrals* is something that needs to be the primary focus of all marketing efforts and forever kept updated.

Frailties of a "usual" medical office "business system"

Henry Ford may have invented the system that revolutionized industrial production speed, but he likely had no idea that his "assembly line" strategy could be used in the business of medical practice.

The purpose of a business system is to maximize the speed, efficiency, productivity, and profitability of business. A business system used in a medical practice business offers the same advantages.

Instead of a medical office full of employees only working jobs that they were hired for, they often have crossover job responsibilities of performing in other job positions when it becomes necessary.

Employees may become ill, have accidents, have family conflicts, or attend special events like graduation ceremonies for a family member, which creates a vacancy of their job position duties in the office. For most medical offices, employees are expected to be knowledgeable enough to do that.

When a job position is suddenly temporarily vacant, another office staff employee is required to do two jobs at the same time (their own and the job of the absent employee).

Efficiency of the office business is immediately diminished because the employee who substitutes is often in a quandary about what the duties are for the person in that position. So they quickly substitute their own ideas about what they think they should do to keep the office functioning. In many cases, the substitute employee lacks knowledge about that job even if he or she has substituted in that job position before.

The great majority of medical offices hire employees who have had some experience in working in other doctor's offices or at least in some kind of office. They are accustomed to using previous experiences and skills form other employments to fill in the gaps of knowledge they need at the time. They have no choice other than to do so.

Private practice doctors rarely take the time to instruct new employees about exactly what their duties are nor how to do them the way the doctor expects them to be done.

After a week or so the new, or substitute, employee has already forgotten the instructions they received, if any were given. It's a mistake every office manager and doctor makes. They never consider that an employee forgets what they're told, which is why they don't keep reminding employees to keep them on track. Francis, the brother of the world-famous marketing expert David Ogilvy, describes this type of dysfunction as "the slippery surface of irrelevant brilliance.

Rarely are new medical office staff members actually taught anything about their new job duties or trained in any way when they are hired; they're just supposed to know. No one there, except the doctor, knows how to do that. As a result, each office staff member does his or her job in a manner that they learned elsewhere or that they think someone (the doctor) wants it to be done.

In this kind of office environment, all a new employee finds out about what they are to do likely was mentioned during their job interview when hired and then forgotten the next day or so.

In addition, and even worse, *99 percent of doctors have no office procedure manuals* that an employee can go to and refresh the details of what they are expected to do in their assigned job position.

When doctors don't have the various office manuals necessary for proper office management available, they are unknowingly exposing themselves to labor lawsuits when they fire an employee and the employee feels they were fired for no legitimate reason, then file a suit.

Usually these litigations end up in favor of the ex-employee because the doctor has no way to back up his or her position without the manuals (and prove that the employee was instructed to read upon being fired) that spell out the details of what an employee can be fired for and how to fire an employee without facing later litigation.

Based on the above information, it's not difficult to understand that a medical office may be in chaos at least half the time, if not all the time. It takes the doctor's time to iron out each management issue when it happens, or maybe only when it gets to the point of scaring all the patients. That wastes time, energy, productivity, and revenue.

Considering what happens in 99 percent of private medical practice offices in terms of the daily operation of the medical business, it's a miracle that medical practices make the income that they do. Beyond that is a vast world of medical practice businesses that continue to function completely independent of the doctor's knowledge, attention, and management. They don't know what they don't know.

If you ask them, the doctors and their employees solidly believe they are functioning at their top capabilities. They might be. But the problem is that those capabilities are not being focused, directed, and coordinated to attain maximum results, efficiency, and productivity.

What all business experts and consultants see going on inside those medical offices is a terribly inefficient business engine barely running on all cylinders. In fact, the lack of their business knowledge prevents them from recognizing all the dysfunctional practices that are losing money for them every single day. When asked how things are going, the doctors and employees most often respond positively about their business progress, which is far from reality.

What do you think happens when a *business-educated physician* starts a private medical practice? At least two-thirds of the usual inefficiency is eliminated, profitability triples, and the well-oiled business engine is humming like a money making machine.

A business system resolves nearly all of these problems in addition to many more dysfunctional issues, and this is how it happens.

The primary goal of the physician's practice must be established by the doctor. That objective is what the whole medical practice business system and series of processes are determined to reach. For example, the doctor may have a desire to increase the number of new patients by 200 percent each month for the next four months. Or maybe the doctor sets eyes on having a million-a-year practice in the next five years.

The big advantage of a "business system" is that it is composed of a *detailed and fixed sequence of "processes"* that each employee is required to follow to maximize their productivity in their job position. They perform the same sequence to complete each job requirement every day. It becomes a habit pattern that can be completed without even thinking about what they should be doing next.

Industry has shown us that doing the same thing the same way every time enables a means of measuring the actual productivity of each employee. Having a way to measure the productivity of medical office staff members to know who is pulling their load and who isn't, is an unknown phenomenon in almost every private practice medical office.

In industry the strict reliance of workers on assembly lines is essential. If one worker sloughs off, the whole line has to slow down or stop. However, in a medical office the system has to be modified to a degree at which the capability of each staff member's job requirements is compatible with maximizing their efficiency and productivity. It means that hiring employees who can handle the job is critical to the accomplishments required by the doctor.

Because the physician is usually the one to hire and fire employees as well as interview new employees, the physician is the one who should create the entire "business system" that covers the detailed series of processes that the physician wants every employee to do in exactly the way the physician wants it done.

This enables the employees to know what the doctor wants done as well as how to do it and leaves no doubt about what they are expected to do. In a way, it's a dictatorship that permits any business to maximize its income and productivity. The problem of an employee wondering about what they are supposed to do and what is expected of them is eliminated.

The medical office adaptation to a business system

The business system in a medical office has to be softened up to be effective. *Employees either make up their own rules to do their jobs* (common in most doctor's offices) or the physician should provide a definite *basic set of rules* for every job duty in their office—at least if they intend to maximize their practice income. (An example of such a list is demonstrated below.)

At the very least it would provide for a smoother running office by eliminating arguments about what employee is responsible for doing what. Mental wrestling matches between employees over who gets to go home first creates anger over having to help other employees finish their jobs at the end of the day so everyone can go home at the same time.

Whining about required overtime at the office and in spite of spouses complaining that the doctor is ruining their family life because of it, is another reason to set the rules when they are hired.

"If you can get yourself to read thirty minutes a day, you're going to double your income every year."
-Brian Tracy

Significant advantages of having a business system.

--Business System Structure--

Example = *Receptionist Duties*

Processes

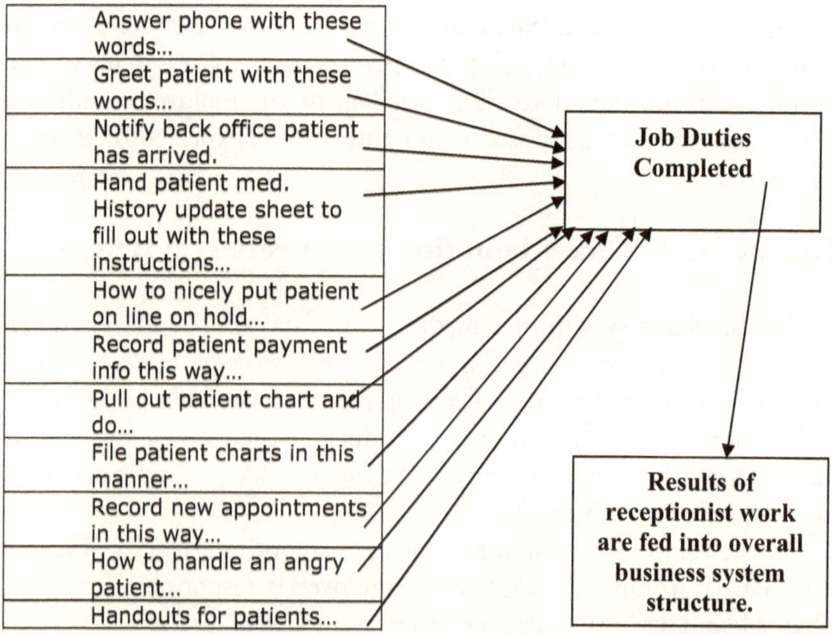

Advantages of a business system:

1. Office projects and goals using a business system can easily be created and added to all the employee's job duties, focus, and attention.

2. Projects and goals can be changed to new ones easily when completed. The system is in place to do it.

3. Team coordination and efforts are inspired repeatedly. What medical office have you seen that works together on specific practice improvement projects?

4. With all job duties already spelled out on paper, all that each employee has to do is shift their attention and focus on the next office improvement process or marketing effort. Some extra job duties may need to be added.

5. Employees discover that their work is more important than they thought and their value to the practice is increased; they feel needed and are more loyal. Their expectation of a salary increase is another stimulating force.

Like an efficient assembly line, the accumulation of the "processes" assigned to each office employee's job position duties becomes the *foundation of the office business system.*

The robotic nature of each process means that each employee knows exactly how to do his or her job step by step for each of his or her assigned duties. All the employee has to do is look at the protocol written on paper or in the office procedures manual and follow each process exactly or are closely as possible.

The advantage of this kind of system is that any employee can be replaced by another with no time lag or loss of productivity. The replacement employee only has to read the detailed step-by-step instructions for that job and ideally step immediately into the job and perform well without a problem.

This is exactly how major industries are able to produce massive amounts of products so quickly and repeatedly. They just plug-in an employee in the production line anywhere they are needed without loss of significant productivity. In a medical office, it has to be done with finesse, persuasively, and gently.

The greatest advantage a business system has for physicians is that, when in place and functional, it will eliminate a significant amount of time spent in managing your medical office.

The doctor's job

1. *Each job position duty* is composed of *multiple step-wise "processes"* that tell the employee exactly how to perform every duty they are assigned.

2. "Multiple processes" created for each job duty assigned and then added to all the job duties of an employee *create a "job system"* for completion of *one job position* in the medical office.

3. *Having multiple "job systems"* for every job position in your medical office added together create the overall *office "business system."*

4. The *total series of "job duty processes"* established for all employee positions is created in such a manner that all processes contribute to the accomplishment of one single objective the doctor has set for the medical practice.

5. The total series of "*job systems*" established for each employee's job position create the *true "business system*" that could be modified, but will never need to be replaced again.

The expected actions taken by each employee done over and over the same way each time is measurable, scalable, easily modifiable, dependable and allows the business system to hum like a well-oiled profit producing machine.

Or would you prefer to continue to spend your time as a physician who's always fixing office and employee problems that intrude on the efficiency and productivity of your medical practice business every day?

What you then have is an organized undercurrent of business chaos that eats away your financial stability and destroys your capacity to improve the primary motivator of your office business—to make enough profit to satisfy you and pay all the bills.

And yes, there is an area of business function between these two extremes that every physician in medical practice can modify to suit the degree of efficiency, profitability, and success that each physician needs to match their own criteria for medical practice business success.

The theme or objective of the business system can be changed anytime to a more focused goal. Goals for medical practices change often for many reasons.

The option remains open to those who have the sagacity and passion to always be improving, expanding, climbing higher, and who are excited about always making progress.

Remember that physicians who create the best business system for their medical practice will always surpass all other physicians who are stuck in the mud of not knowing how to get out of the inertia that shackles them.

Lesson: Until the medical education elite decide, not just think about, to include a formal business education for all medical students, the academic medical school system will continue to graduate *wounded doctors* whose business wounds never heal.

Those who are predestined to fail are sadly left lying on the medical practice business battlefield. And it certainly accounts for the attrition of physicians and the deterioration of the medical profession in a business world today that demands business knowledge to survive. Why is that so hard to see?

Other important requirements associated with smoothly running and efficient medical office businesses are often overlooked, such as...

1. Every employee must be comfortable with working as a team member. Knowing how to select such people is another learning process. Those who turn out not to be teamwork oriented should be quickly replaced.

2. Every employee has to be well informed about the primary goal or goals of the physician, not the "manager" of the practice, if other than the doctor.

3. Each employee must understand his or her position in the business system and what is expected of him or her. This highlights the importance of the list of "processes" written down in detail for them to follow.

4. After being created, the business system machine must be continually oiled and greased to remain functional. Oversight and correction of blunders must be handled carefully so as not to reduce the creativity of each employee. It's another management skill that physicians often will only learn during a business education endeavor.

5. To improve or just maintain the motivation, energy, and creative flow of employees, it's necessary to provide them with frequent progress reports, refocusing on the objectives, supervision, and respect for their work in the system. There are good and bad ways to do that.

6. Remembering that each employee is naturally working towards their *own objectives, not the doctor's goals*. This is done by making them aware of the increased benefits they will receive when they pitch in and do a great job to enhance the office and medical business functions. Often, the benefits are the same as what the employee already has in mind.

The thought that there are more benefits than they expected in performing their job is always an effective stimulus for loyalty to the cause.

7. Business management always involves people, as everyone knows. What most managers don't know is how to trigger each employee's magic button. You know, the one that instantly inspires them to perform better. Every person has a different trigger mechanism so it takes time for most doctors to find the right one to use.

   Office business managers also need to know how to uncover the triggers that work with each employee. Sometimes it's praise for a job well done. For others it's a salary increase. Many respond to being allowed to show their creativity in their job. When those triggers are discovered, almost everyone is vulnerable to being led to achieve better goals and higher performance.

   Over the long haul the time spent managing these things is far less than the time spent repairing problems caused by the absence of a business system. That results in less productivity and business income.

   The crushing thing about the business of medical practice that seems to be universal is that nearly all physicians come to believe that what they have settled for in their medical practice is *all they can hope for* in their future. They don't know what they don't know. They have no idea what they are really capable of doing with the right business tools.

   A formal business education opens their eyes to what they can accomplish in their medical practice career by the full implementation of their business knowledge and business tools. It's shocking for them to understand there's so much more to be had that they would otherwise never have recognized.

   You may have even chuckled to yourself when President Kennedy said in 1962 he was going to put a man on the moon by 1969. Space travel at the time was something most people believed to be impossible, at least not for another century. The fact that it was done inspired everyone on earth, it seemed, to greater achievement and new possibilities formerly considered a pipedream.

I believe that same exhilarating and inspirational effect will be as profound for each and every physician in private medical practice when they experience the medical practice opportunities that a formal business education will give them. The dimension it will add to the medical profession and every physician will be nothing short of overwhelming. (Please re-read that last paragraph over again.)

"You have absolute control over but one thing: your thoughts. This divine prerogative is the sole means by which you may control your destiny. If you fail to control your mind, you will control nothing else. Your mind is your spiritual estate. What you hold in your mind today will shape your experiences of tomorrow."

---Napoleon Hill, author of "Think and Grow Rich"

Please Note: Free copy of this iconic eBook is available to you on my website.

CHAPTER 8

The Treatment Plan

"The Essentials Required for Creating a Formal Business Education for All Medical Students are Urgent, Necessary, and Incredibly Beneficial to All Participants"

There's adequate reason to believe and trust that medical schools have the sagacity and capacity to create a formal business education program for medical students that will dramatically improve the capacity of every physician in private medical practice to reach their maximum potential while serving the expanding medical needs of our country, even the world.

Alternatives, proposed basics, and administration of such an academic business education of all medical students.

1. Pros and cons of a "voluntary" business education program.

ADVANTAGEOUS BENEFITS OCCUR with both. Between them a hybrid model could be created, which could focus on delivering a tailored business education to a segmented group of medical students. Such a segmented group could be created by a voluntary request from them for a formal business education during their normal medical school curriculum.

The great difficulty with that arrangement likely would be trying to persuade beginning medical students that a formal business education is essential to their private practice of medicine. The difficulty of recruiting student volunteers would be comparable to trying to persuade children to learn how to swim when they have never been in a swimming pool before.

Logically, such volunteers would already have to be knowledgeable about the facts, details, risks, consequences, and security of such a new area of education to make a decision to volunteer themselves into such a supplemental business program.

The business education program created should be appropriate for their career goals in private medical practice and not oriented to a life of an employed physician where business is done for them.

Creating a hybrid model is extravagant and unnecessary when one considers the cost, administration of, and constant updating of such a program for so few students who might volunteer to be included.

A class survey would be especially important for all medical students who already have been told about the widely known and abundant advantages that business knowledge provides their medical careers. If *students have no idea* what a business education can do for them, a survey would be useless.

One exception might be to compare the overall medical student interest in such a business education when one group with "cold" knowledge (what previous knowledge they carry from college-premed into medical school) can be compared to another group who has already been fully educated about the known advantages for any physician in private medical practice.

It would be expected that most students would be interested if they understand the great advantage that an academic business education can provide any physician in private medical practice.

The likelihood of the massive voluntary participation of nearly every medical student in the business education process might be predictable. It's based on their expected behavior when classmate competition is involved.

No student wants to miss out on an incredible opportunity that might profoundly benefit them in their medical career, especially when other classmates appear to already know the great value being offered—and they don't.

Some important advantages of voluntary participation are:

1. Students would be able to access business education materials anytime at their own convenience during the full duration of their four-year medical education studies.

2. The gathering of business knowledge and study is the complete responsibility of the student (in this scenario).

3. Students would not be restricted by requirements regarding the amount of time spent on the business learning nor on the depth of learning they accomplish.

   It would be of value to have a series of tests available for students to take voluntarily and could be used to test their business knowledge level. Test results are an excellent means of evaluating how effective such a voluntary business learning process is. Just as important is to discover what teaching methods and presentations produce the best student-testing results.

   The testing process is one good means of discovering how to improve the business education structure, teaching points, value to students, and lecture content and delivery.

4. A manual or syllabus that would have a systematic guide for students to follow should be available. As with any learning course, there's a proper educational sequence for learning any topic that makes it much easier to learn, remember, and refer back to at any time.

5. The best formats for business education in today's environment would be CDs, DVDs, online lecture series, business online webinars and teleseminars, suggested lists of business educational resources to read, watch (videos), or use, such as references to specific priority of books, videos, business education articles and other business publications.

   There are enormous numbers of resources online today that are about business education and are available for free. The validity and educational value of these resources would have to be reviewed and meet the standards established by the course educators.

6. Live lecture series on business principles can be presented at convenient times for students so as not to interfere with the regular medical education curriculum. Early evenings, weekends, noon-times, and during holiday breaks would be the most obvious times. Some medical schools offer a fifth year of school for comparable educational reasons.

   A live lecture series given by well-known business experts and public educational speakers would eventually become an added feature of the business education curriculum once the preliminary business education strategies and tactics prove to be effective learning tools.

7. The business materials should be available 24/7 (if possible) throughout the full four years of the standard medical school curriculum. It would allow adequate time for any student to learn what they will need to know (at least the basics) to run their medical practice business more efficiently and profitably.

2. Pros and cons of "required" student participation

Taking into consideration the common beliefs and behavioral patterns of students who are told that the business course is voluntary or free of charge sends them *four detrimental subliminal messages that tend to discourage student participation*:

1. If it's voluntary, it's of little value.

2. If it's free, it's of little or no value.

3. If it's additional learning on top of an already busy academic schedule, no thanks.

4. If it's **not** directly associated with or part of the "medical" education process, forget it.

These four issues are enough to convince anyone that making business education a required course is *mandatory*. Why would a medical school go to the trouble of creating a formal business education course if only thirty students out of a class of one hundred sixty-five would volunteer to take the course in the first place?

Once a dozen or so of the students who actually take the course start bragging about how much they have learned about marketing and business related to medical practice, especially to those classmates who rejected the course, what is your guess about what would happen as a result?

One can never be 100 percent sure, but there is little doubt that the great majority, if not all of the class would not only develop a severe case of "missing-out-itis" on an exclusive opportunity of great value to them, but would also quickly ignite a stampede to sign-up for the business course, simply because of their embarrassment in seeing that a large group of other students were able to anticipate the value of a business education before they did, and that would be hard to swallow.

It's a time, cost, and value issue for any medical school.

A second factor, and even more supportive of business education being required, is the fact that medical students have no idea how important business knowledge will be when they start their medical practice. It has to be taught to them, and they will begin to appreciate the value and the importance of it later.

The same pattern exists for the medical school curriculum as well. No student really knows the full importance of what they are being taught medically until after they graduate and begin to use it.

"The quality of a person's life is in proportion to their commitment to excellence regardless of their chosen field of endeavor."
-Vince Lombardi

Some important aspects of *required* participation

1. The educational process is prearranged by means of a structured course curriculum scheduled into appropriate times available to the majority of students who will attend.

The business curriculum can be run in repeat loop cycles during the four-year educational stint, so that all students can get access to what they missed or have forgotten in the previous cycles.

By taking note of the suggested business topics that every student should have a reasonable grasp of (listed below), it would be possible to cycle the compete business education curriculum about three times while a student travels through the four-year medical school system.

There are many ways to readjust the business course to match the space allowed by the institution and medical education priorities.

2. All digital and written education materials would be made available to students 24/7 for review and learning.

3. Live lecture series on various aspects of business should be scheduled at times when most of the students are free to attend. When the series ends, the series starts over again.

   Live presentations are much more effective for many reasons. For example, a direct Q and A period at the end of the lecture can't be reproduced as effectively in any other manner later.

   This Q and A process offers a great feedback mechanism for lecturers to understand the predominant concerns of the audience. The lecturer can then improve on the presentation in the future.

   The Q and A segment in reality is a continuation of (but informal) the educational process available to any or all students and tends to be highly attractive to students with inquisitive minds and those who are able to perceive that there just might well be a field of diamonds hidden within their grasp.

4. When a course is "required," it sends a message to students that a business education is just as important to their medical careers as medical education. It's a fact that hopefully may irritate a significant number of medical educators enough to incite action.

5. The business course will and should involve giving tests to students to evaluate the strength and weaknesses of their learning the information and to evaluate the course materials and lectures that are not up to par, and need improvement.

6. The lecturers' can be "borrowed" from the *business school's staff* or from *senior business school students*, when available.

   Hiring outside business experts, which I recommend, is also a brilliant option. This means those who have reached and maintained their ultimate business success by earning that distinction the hard way: by experiencing the hard knocks and challenges, while the possibility of failure shadows them along the way.

   Doing it while suffering setbacks and failures along the way adds something to a student's business education that can't be duplicated by business professors in the college classroom. It's often a criticism made about the MBA classroom programs.

   Medical school staff and instructors, being raised in the medical profession without a formal business education themselves are not truly qualified to teach a business course, at least in my experience.

7. *Live business education lectures* can be recorded (DVDs, CDs, video, and podcasts) and made available to students who missed the lectures.

   These recordings can also be sold to other professional schools as a means of funding the business education curriculum.

   When all live lectures have been recorded in a business course series, then *further live lectures* would not be needed for a period of time after.

   When there are new updates and changes to be made in the business education course, a new live lecture is warranted, then recorded and used in place of the outdated materials.

8. The permanent "business education position" of the *business education coordinator* at the medical school should be a highly qualified and experienced person in the field of education curriculums. Those individuals can be recruited from such organizations as **Coursera.**

(All salient touchstones have not been included as you can see, but are no less important than those listed immediately above. Check the references at the end of this book.)

It's my belief that the reason medical school academics and scholars have avoided this business education responsibility so long is they don't have the business knowledge to understand everything such education offers.

3. The timing, content, and positioning factors relating to a business education course.

Options for inserting business education into the medical education curriculum will vary from school to school depending on their priorities, available time, and decisions arrived at that reflect their level of commitment.

The commitment is to graduate medical doctors with the knowledge, education, and capability to reach their maximum medical and career potential, which can only be attained by the combination of business and medical education together.

The factors that validate this conclusion are described in this treatise.

Some of those options are:

A. The business course should include *about sixty live lectures* and should be scheduled once a week at the same time and place every week that is most appropriate and available to all medical students.

B. An adequate business education will require *at least sixty featured pillars of business knowledge* that can be made available to students in one of many ways as mentioned earlier in this chapter.

C. A suggested list of business (includes marketing) education knowledge topics likely to be included in the business education of medical students:

(not listed in order of priority, educational sequence, or intrinsic content and educational value—each contains valuable business lessons that are normally focused on a specific important segment of business knowledge.)

1. Why a business education is important to all physicians
2. The effects and value of business knowledge in medical practice
3. Reasons for calling a medical practice a business and then not treating it as one.
4. Who's responsible for providing the business education… medical schools, medical students, or others?
5. The problems associated with practicing medicine with no formal business education
6. The factors that determine the success or failure of the business of medical practice.
7. What doctors need to know about business and why
8. The full meaning, understanding, and use of marketing
9. The difference between marketing and advertising
10. Importance of copywriting in the medical business world
11. How to write an ad for your medical practice.
12. How marketing benefits a medical practice business and other businesses
13. Various forms or kinds of current marketing methods
14. Current best and worst marketing methods for physicians

15. Costs of various marketing methods

16. How a physician's attitude and goals makes a difference in the method of marketing used

17. How to measure the effectiveness of your marketing method.

18. How to construct a marketing strategy.

19. How to construct a business plan.

20. Value and use of a medical practice website

21. Value and use of social media

22. Various forms and use of media in marketing strategies

23. How to use persuasion tactics with patients

24. How to use your patients to promote your medical practice for you

25. How to create and maintain an efficient referral program from other doctors

26. Techniques for promoting your own practice

27. How to create a medical practice website and manage it

28. The best use of a medical website

29. How to use social media sites to market your practice

30. The serious risks to your business caused by any medical malpractice litigation.

31. How to create a marketing plan

32. The critical importance of having goals

33. How the selection of a place to practice will help or hinder your future practice success

34. How to work smart, not hard, in medical practice

35. The importance of "follow-up" in marketing your practice

36. The essential rules for hiring and firing employees

37. How to persuade your office employees to promote your medical practice

38. How to magnify your customer service efforts to increase the loyalty of your patients

39. The important relationship between marketing and the amount of funds you allocate to it

40. Why physicians abhor marketing and management of their medical practice business—and ways to change that attitude

41. Why being the first to do anything always places a doctor at the forefront in the eyes of potential patients

42. What a medical practice newsletter can do for your medical practice and how to start one

43. How to publish and distribute a well-received newsletter for your patients

44. How to do marketing for attracting new patients

45. How to create a highly effective business card that is rarely thrown away

46. The importance of having your own printed medical information handouts for your patients and using them for your marketing

47. Causes of medical practice financial failure

48. Serious reasons for moving your medical practice and when to do it

49. How to outsource segments of your office practice business

50. The importance of understanding the reasons for continued practice marketing efforts

51. How to know if your medical practice is failing

52. How to survey your patients and get them to respond well

53. How to bring back patients that left your practice

54. How to build trust in your patients for your medical services and advice

55. Ways to prevent a medical or surgical error from becoming a malpractice suit

56. The importance of saying "thank you" as a marketing ploy and doing it effectively

57. About the value of marketing and business knowledge if you decide to change careers or have to leave your medical practice for some reason

58. The advantages of having business and marketing knowledge if you join a private medical practice group practice

59. The serious consequences of running a medical practice business with no business or marketing education

60. Why you shouldn't ever retire from medical practice voluntarily

4. The realities and practicalities of a business education for medical students.

The most productive physicians reach their maximum potential only when they have the mindset to do so. Their mindset is most often the result of the visualization process in the mind's eye as to what they imagine their future to be and is supported and perpetuated by an unrelenting determination to reach their maximum potential.

In reality many medical students for whatever reasons don't have the tenacity, drive, or determination to do much more than become a regular medical doctor and level off there. Some of the most important reasons seem to be related to factors that are either attributed to dissatisfaction with their career choice or to their psychological makeup.

Students level off primarily because of "educational" burnout, something that isn't talked about much. Their vision and destination over all those years in preparation for medical school graduation was to become a regular medical doctor, not a *fantastic* medical doctor.

It's a new way of thinking about and then initiating their "second generation" of personal commitment, an invigoration of new passion, and the firing-up of their self-discipline and determination to make it happen.

Added to the decrease of passion to extend themselves to higher accomplishments is the overwhelming urge to start practicing medicine that every physician has been dreaming about for years and the wait necessary to get started. It seems that their passion isn't really decreased, but is transferred to another priority in their career path that is more important to them at the time.

Although the necessity of paying off educational debts lies in the background, young doctors may see that as a reason to forget specialty training if possible and jump into an employed position with the guarantee of a paycheck twice a month.

The disturbing thought of living in relative poverty as a private practice physician for many more years frequently counters all present goals and passions of medical doctors.

How one might be able to persuade medical students to create a mindset for future higher goals rather than to service their career at a "less-than-full capability" level.

Having choices and options open to them that they have not thought about is a good place to start. Obtaining a good business education is one of them. It may be that getting that business education will have to be delayed forever if they are forced to do it themselves. That's why obtaining it while they are still medical students is important and is the right time for it.

With the additional business education background, students are much more open-minded about decisions to add specialty training to their skills, knowledge, and capabilities.

Business education increases their self-esteem, magnifies their responsibility, improves their feelings about career security, and, most importantly, boosts their self-confidence and belief that they are truly capable of doing more in their career than they ever imagined.

That's because they will come to understand that the increase in medical skills and knowledge, when founded on a strong business foundation and business principles, will empower them to recognize that they can move to higher levels in practice, income, and productivity.

They already have the two inborn skills instead of just one that can push *possibilities* up to *probabilities*, but often never recognize them.

1. **A decisive entrepreneurial spirit that most students and doctors really don't recognize in themselves**

2. **The ability to see their true purpose in life that goes far beyond what parents demand of them and what they have previously demanded of themselves**

Another choice for opening up their visualization of their potential in medical practice would be for medical schools to routinely allow students during their "elective times" to do apprenticeships with practicing doctors locally, as this author did and knows of its value to future medical practice decisions and mindset. Some medical schools already provide these opportunities.

Other possibilities can be experimented with. You want students to look at their world beyond medical school graduation with fresh eyes and rejuvenated passion. It can be done. When you're leading the race and can see the finish line ahead, that same surge of passion and desire is the same feeling and emotion one needs here.

A business education for all medical students is a highly profitable investment that medical schools should make to achieve the benefits derived from smarter and more confident graduates who are eager to praise their school and give back to the school in many more ways.

"There are both logical and justifiable reasons for medical education academics to want to participate in efforts to save private medical practice from complete disintegration.

There are logical and justifiable reasons for medical education academics to join in efforts to prevent doctors from facing the medical practice and career destroying epidemic of *business ignorance* that lies at the core of private medical practice physician frustration today.

There are logical and justifiable reasons for implementing an academic business education of all medical students today.

There are NO logical and justifiable reasons for medical schools to continue their disregard of a business education for medical students... especially in light of increasing financial failures of medical practices, increasing attrition of physicians, and overwhelming frustrations that all doctors today feel when they learn that medical schools may have intentionally betrayed their trust."

5. The earlier a business mentality enters the mind, the greater will be the medical student's acceptance of a business education.

When the mind is young, fresh, and eager for knowledge and before the barriers concerning the need for business knowledge are created, the *business mind-set* can be firmly established. The business nature of man is a natural instinct, but has to be intentionally cultivated for its most advantageous and perpetual rewards.

Much has been written about this, and there is no doubt that the encouragement of teenagers, even much younger kids, to start a business of their own and run it themselves would be a welcome and tremendous asset to them later.

Children are quite able start a business even earlier than eight years old with the proper parental or mentor encouragement and instruction. Direct motivation and stimulation by parents or other family members is required. The minds of children are easily distracted, so a focus on the importance of business to them at an early age is paramount to their satisfaction with their later careers in medicine.

With the advent of the Internet and its level playing field for business startups, many teenage millionaires as well as college student millionaires are often being reported in the media. The opportunities for doing this are escalating.

Many young people are now able to pay for their own college and graduate education with the profits from their own businesses. Young people's financial freedom is critical to the financial survival of parents who are shackled with the educational debt accumulated by paying for their children's education.

Any child or teenager with the right talents and desires, when encouraged and mentored by parents (or a trusted adult, such as Robert Kiyosaki, author, business millionaire who has created such a program for kids), can learn business principles, use them effectively, and have no limitation to their capabilities.

Not only does this manner of developing a business mind at an early age while headed for the medical professional life and career give them a leg up on all other medical students, but also over all other physicians with no significant prior business education and experience.

Medical scholars commonly find that medical students with a formal business education and business experience prior to medical school rise to the top of the medical education game much faster. They also have the business competence to be far more successful than most physicians.

This is a factor that should be part of any premedical curriculum guidance today.

A classmate of mine in medical school had previously worked ten years in the U.S. State Department. He had the maturity, qualities, and communication skills we all needed but didn't have. These factors were quickly recognized and he was elected class president all four years, to our great advantage.

Another classmate of mine, the late Henry Jordan, MD, is the best example of a business-educated and business-minded medical professional I have ever befriended. His business acumen at the University of Pennsylvania, Perelman School of Medicine established an educational legacy that will be hard to surpass. This book I consider to be worthy of honoring Dr. Jordan's business education accomplishments at the School Of Medicine.

Now, if these two examples don't demonstrate the power of a business background and knowledge and the influence they have on the ultimate professional success of all physicians today, then tell me what will.

If you truly believe that a business education is not necessary for medical students or doctors, then it should behoove you to start a medical practice without any form of business foundation.

If any physician today has not yet started on a project at home to stimulate, teach, and encourage his or her young children to understand the use of money, understand business principles, and generate the desire to learn about the advantages of business education, then shame on you.

If you desire to balance your professional career demands with your home life and family, then this is what you, at the very least, should be doing. But getting your children to start their own business is even better.

**"Without involvement, there is no commitment.
Mark it down, asterisk it, circle it, underline it.
No involvement, no commitment."**
-Stephen Covey

6. Responsibility for premedical student preparation regarding business education while in "college."

The prevailing idea that every *premed student* should receive a well-rounded education is outdated, if not a hindrance to the later medical student's eventual success in their medical career. If college premeds started by reading a national newspaper, like the *Wall Street Journal*, daily throughout college years, it would be a formidable start towards their well-rounded practical business education. Add to that a subscription to the Harvard Business News and newsletter.

With the increasing demand on time management in this world of overpowering access to knowledge it's necessary for education to be highly streamlined, more focused, and highly supportive of the essential knowledge required for professional career success.

The dental profession, for example, has survived the short three-year college requirement for acceptance into dental school and now has at less educational cost created more millionaire dentists than ever before. Medical schools could do the same and not compromise the quality of the medical profession. It's a profound testimonial for shortening premed education in college.

When you think about it, premeds apply for and are accepted to medical schools based on their first three years of college education, not the fourth year that they have yet to complete. Medical schools will hopefully come around to their senses eventually. The old adage that premedical students need that fourth year to mature before beginning medical school is inappropriate, unnecessary, and is obsolete today.

The Jefferson University Medical School in Philadelphia a generation ago accepted students who were gifted enough to meet the demands of medical education regardless of age, amount of college education, or lack of required curriculum courses. They proved it works well and produced good doctors. Yet the general drift of requirements for admission remains the same as ever among most medical schools. Why?

Along with that is the fact that we grow up faster, mature quicker, and have the educational and technological capabilities that far exceed previous generations at the same ages.

With all these factors and others, it becomes evident that premed curriculums should be required to focus on delivering a premedical student to medical school that *understands business principles.* Simply understanding that business knowledge has a profound effect on the level of success of any business is a great beginning. Undergraduate education today is structured to help graduates *get a job, not a career.*

Having a job for half of a lifetime rarely offers any employee much more than a bump in salary or position, certainly not security or opportunity.

When business knowledge is added to almost any career you can name, success is not a matter of "if," but a matter of "how much."

Serious premed students will "get it" but still need guidance on selecting business courses or topics appropriate for medical practice such as:

1. National economic changes that occur often and business changes that need to be made to remain financially stable in any business

2. A thorough exploration of the actual business elements that make or break a medical practice business, or any business

3. The power of a business education to favorably alter the careers of any professional, including medical doctors

4. How to manage money in business, the value of financial statements, and what they can tell you

5. The profit value of marketing

6. How business and marketing strategies are used to resolve financial problems

This kind of preparation will result in remarkable benefits to any college premed student, whether they are accepted to medical school or not. But it certainly improves their qualifications for entrance.

In my estimation, the majority of premed programs in colleges require a much more intensive and focused effort to dramatically improve requirements for their premed students to stay in the premed program. Perhaps requirements to even qualify to apply to medical school should be in order.

> **There is no significant downside to an academic business education. In one way or another it affects the way we live our lives and provides opportunities that otherwise will be lost.**

Why not advise students to get an MBA after college graduation or immediately after medical school graduation?

Reasons why it's *not* a good plan are:

1. Interruption in the progress of a passionate endeavor is known to destroy passion and desire for attaining that objective later.

2. The standard academic curriculum required for a Masters in Business Administration at most academic institutions today is too generalized in business knowledge content to be of significant help for a *physician in private medical practice.* However, it's better than no business education at all.

3. An MBA degree costs on average from $20,000 to $40,000 for a two-year on-campus academic program. Adding this fee to that of the medical education means a total of around $200,000, which is not affordable for most students even with scholarship aid.

4. The usual MBA program would have to be drastically modified to meet the needs of most medical doctors whose primary ambition is to practice medicine and to learn how to manage a medical practice business.

5. Doctors, dentists, and lawyers are a different breed of professionals that require a much more focused and relevant business education.

The business education of doctors has to be presented in a manner that is closely connected to and intertwined with the business factors in medical practice.

To be meaningful enough for medical students to easily understand how business strategies and principles fit together with a busy office medical practice, all have to be directly *associated with a medical practice business problem and solution.*

By bonding the business solutions tightly to the practice business problems, any student can clearly see their business education as an integral part of the medical practice structure and not an entity that is separate in nature and has to be brought in and fitted into medical practice business.

The perfect time to accomplish that is when medical students learn both business and medicine together. It psychologically locks the mixture together as a mindset that should be expected to last throughout their medical career.

If medical schools and academic medicine scholars never intend to have anything to do with providing a business education to medical students, there are viable alternatives for them. Many updated MBA curriculums have been introduced online. Many of these MBA programs have purposely been shortened to a year in length which is a great advantage to young doctors.

Hybrid MBA programs have been created, like the STAR program at George Washington University in D.C. for professional athletes who have been forced out of professional sports. The typical story is that they spent all of their earnings with no plan for the future and were financially broke when forced out. It's a do-it-at-home program while they work in a job.

The business education above is unique because one can perform the necessary learning at home while also working at a job. It requires intermittently attending the program at the school along the way to meet the learning standards.

This type of program will likely become available to other professionals, including doctors, as education is turning to online learning for those who can't afford a full time on-campus business education. That will enable doctors to get a business education while continuing to practice medicine. The major drawback is the proven fact that most all doctors won't acquire a business education once they are in private practice.

The business education will be the solution to the one formidable barrier that prevents practicing physicians from obtaining such a necessary area of knowledge. Practicing physicians refuse to take time away from their practices, and loss of income while they are away, to get a business education on their own. You can't blame them for making that decision.

The documented fact that the physicians will rarely, if ever, voluntarily take the time and pay the price for an academic business education, lends indisputable support for the idea of providing the business knowledge during medical school.

A real life example of the value and importance of a business education for medical students

A recent experience I had with a second-year medical student confirmed my thoughts about several factors relating to what a good business education offers to medical students. This student with a college and an MBA degree introduced himself by sending me an email to thank me for my ***Advanced Medical Practice Business and Marketing E-zine Newsletter*** he had subscribed to.

What he found to be especially valuable to himself were my articles (over sixty on my website) dedicated to educating medical students and physicians about the business issues of importance to private medical practice. Because he was well versed about business and marketing already, he was able to easily understand the way that I connected business issues to the actual practice of medicine.

He explained to me that for the first time in his college and medical school education, he had found a resource that honestly applied business principles to real medical practice in detail, with strategies to use, the explanations for use of each and every element of marketing, and the reasons every medical student should have this business knowledge.

What to me has been the most satisfying aspect of our communications over the last two years is that this was the first communication from a medical student over the last six years that my articles have been online for anyone to read and learn, and it came from a student with a prior academic business education.

It showed me that a new medical student already understood the importance of business to the success level of every business, including medical practice, and clearly understood the critical value of a business education for doctors from his view inside of the profession.

It points out what I alluded to several pages above about the necessity to teach medical students and premed students what a business education can do for them in their medical practice, before it's possible to persuade them to obtain a formal business education in spite of the cost.

This experience incited me to create a website specifically for medical students to learn about business and marketing early in their careers. The URL address: www.MedicalStudentTips.com. The site also contains information and advice relating to problems and solutions for medical practice that are never taught in medical school and will help students stay out of trouble while in medical practice.

"The only unpardonable sin of any living thing, beast or man, is attempting to stay "as is" for very long."
-Robert Collier

Ideas about how to persuade medical students to follow advice and recommendations about business education that seem contrary to their normal expectations are...

One Sunday a few weeks ago a young pastor gave a talk on TV about "Follow Me" which fits this discussion we are having, and I'd like you to think of it as a technique for persuading medical students to commit wholeheartedly to a formal business education.

My wife and I have developed a routine on Sunday morning of viewing helpful family and business programs online. Aside from our Bible reading, many online programs provide an opportunity to learn about family and business issues and their solutions.

These programs are usually about human communication issues but are exemplified by problems in marriage, politics, government, personal issues, and the importance of faith in our lives. Frequently, these are lessons that are applicable to *everyday living and business life.* You don't have to be a Christian to watch and learn. They are valuable ideas and solutions that anyone can listen to and use to improve their own lives or businesses.

One of these educators is a young man who is able to connect life and business lessons to the Biblical teachings much better than most. His presentation technique is unique and easy to remember.

Although pastor Andy Stanley's presentation (you can find him on "YouTube" by searching ("Pastor Andy Stanley") from the stage is informal and he walks around on the stage and uses a slide/screen assistant. It's not any different than most other college or public lectures I've attended in my life. His focus was on four major sequential steps to create the behavior.

Four sequential processes create a predictable behavior. (Adapted to the need for a business education)

(These are applicable to any religion, any form of belief, and to those without religious beliefs.)

1. **Sit and listen:** This process is one of getting a student's attention first. When Christ began recruiting his disciples, he simply said, "Follow me." There was no recruitment speech given, no pressure to leave everything, no threats if they didn't follow, no packing up, and no warnings about what would happen if they refused.

   So why did each of the twelve disciples just stop what they were doing at the time without one word of objection and follow him (according to the Bible)?

   What Christ did was spend time talking to all those listening about how to improve their lives in a manner quite different from what they had always been hearing.

   Tactic: It opens the mind and stimulates interest when the audience understands how the issue will positively affect their lives. It's one of the most effective marketing tactics used today—straight from the Bible.

2. **Correct information:** Jesus told those who were interested in finding out how to find personal satisfaction with their lives how to do it.

   But to believe it, one has to trust the source of the information as well as the promise being made. Trust of a person comes from a spotless prior reputation for doing what they say they will do (called integrity), and the truth of what's being told is always confirmed later.

   Trust is also a perception created by the way it's presented, the words and how they're used, and the sincerity of the person who is speaking.

   People need to understand how to process the information into what value it may have for them.

   It's not enough to tell the listening audience (or patient) about your product or ideas that you think they might like or buy into. Persuasion results from presenting the information that this audience wants at this time, in this place, under these conditions, is exactly what they are seeking answers for.

   Tactic: People have an uncanny way of recognizing B.S. when they hear or read it. When the right information is being handed out to the right people who need that information, it's interpreted as being a one-on-one conversation. It sets up further belief in what is said and primes the acceptance of the next step in the process.

3. **Documentation:** Jesus never paid the disciples for their work that he instructed them to do. No obligation to Christ was made by the disciples, so they could have quit at any time—but never did, which is an unbelievable circumstance.

   For the disciples to be completely persuaded to do what Christ wanted, it was necessary to teach them and show them the power of faith by demonstrating what it can accomplish.

   The miracles he performed with healing people, raising the dead, and feeding ten thousand at one time with three fishes and two or three loaves of bread were real to everyone who witnessed such happenings.

Tactic: This is the level at which a person's decision is made. Showing customers that a product or service (medical practice) does what it is supposed to do and keeps doing it repeatedly is always convincing. It's why a free trial of a product is offered and a guarantee is given to return your payment if you are not satisfied.

The percentage return rates for purchased commercial items are about 1-3 percent. If it rises to 10 percent, the sales company has a serious problem. The same factors are true for a medical practice as well. Suppose one in every ten patients left your practice: a very good reason to keep logs on new and old patients.

4. **Follow the advice:** People need to prove to themselves that doing what they are told and advised to do, is safe, has value to them and can be a formidable benefit to them and others when taken advantage of.

   The final step for persuading twelve complete strangers (disciples) of various professions, from various economic levels of society, and with no reason to work without pay, can't really be explained, but it worked. The disciples had to take action and perform as expected—another unexplainable enigma.

Tactic: Medical patients and store customers have decided to buy into the process at this point, but it will never happen until they keep their first medical office appointment or fork over the money to buy the product.

Once a customer touches the product, uses it, and it works, marketers know that over 90 percent of buyers will not return the product nor ask for their money back, even if they find a couple minor troubling issues. It's the same with medical patients.

It takes about six visits to their new medical doctor for patients to completely trust their doctor. It happens to be the same number of contacts that need to be made with a customer before they trust the salesperson, the product, or service enough to buy the product or service.

I chose this way of explaining behavior in a simple way. How much and how often we have predictable behavior patterns that were present even two thousand years ago, is unknown. It's a good example of how and why most medical students will choose to accept, and maybe even demand, a business education after implementing these tactics.

What is remarkable is that the living God and Christ performed a feat with the recruitment of twelve disciples that remains an enigma to this day.

Enigma or not, it works!

"Real persuasion comes from putting more of you into everything you say. Words have an effect. Words loaded with emotion have a powerful effect."
-Jim Rohn

CHAPTER 9

The Cost of Treatment

"Options for How Medical Schools can Fund an Academic Business Education for All Medical Students"

(After medical schools are able to overcome their discriminatory objections to providing an academic business education for medical students, it will inevitably revolutionize the medical profession stability and quality.)

Many reasonable resources are available today for funding such a critically important project that has been neglected far too long.

CONTRARY TO WHAT you may believe, there is no shortage of money in our nation. One simply has to know where it is and how to get it.

As we all know, it makes good business sense to establish and secure sources for funding before presenting a business education course for approval.

Knowing that there already is a fully active curriculum for the medical education of students, there is an option to add this business education project to the existing medical school curriculum and avoid creating another separate education plan.

The ultimate decision to implement a business education curriculum into the medical curriculum will be at the discretion of decision-makers with entrepreneurial minds. I refer to those who actually understand and believe in the overwhelming benefit of such an undertaking to every element of the medical education system nationwide.

This one undertaking will prevent the tsunami of physician attrition we see today, because the root origin of the problem of attrition is *money*. When physicians know how to earn the money they will be satisfied with in medical practice, 99 percent of doctor attrition will disappear automatically.

No longer will the widespread increasing frustration among physicians about medical practice inadequacy (which is really the lack of adequate production of income) be the leading cause of the attrition.

Who doesn't understand this indisputable connection?

Ultimately, no medical doctor will remain in medical practice when their monetary compensation is inadequate for their status, education, and value to the nation, regardless of their passion for the practice of medicine and their dedication to helping the ill and injured patients.

Apparently, there is a majority of medical professional education scholars who don't recognize the full cost associated with the commoditization of physician professionals who are overworked and underpaid in today's marketplace.

When a physician has earned the distinction of being called a doctor, medical doctor, or physician, that physician should be honored as such in the media, by authorities outside of medicine and medical practice, and removed from the generic terminology labeling used today—"healthcare provider."

It's another cultural and progressive ideology for intimidation of physicians that author Robert Ringer should write another book about.

Would anyone be surprised to hear at the annual medical school graduation ceremonies, "This medical school is honored and delighted to present graduation certificates to another class of elite 'healthcare providers' and doctor certificates will indicate such a distinguished title for the world to recognize."

Some well-known alternatives for funding and other support that can be viable opportunities are:

1. Physician alumni who donate money to their medical school

2. Outside donations from organizations or anonymous people

3. Medical companies that support physician education, such as pharmaceutical companies, charitable foundations, research organizations, government grants, private solicited wealthy donors with a healthcare improvement incentive, etc.

4. Countries or organizations outside the USA that send their students to the USA for their education, particularly medical education

5. Shared financial resources that are available to the majority of medical schools, yet not being used presently to any accessible degree

6. Medical students who agree to pay for their business education while in medical school, with the amount to be set by the school administration decision makers

7. Diversion of segments of large monetary donations made towards other purposes or for implementing business education as an integral related part of the purpose they were originally intended for

8. Crowdfunding, venture capital, and other resources that you know of, and I'm not aware of.

Resources for funding are available even in a down economy. Reliance on the creativeness, ingenuity, and entrepreneurial ingredients of a few dedicated people is all it takes for one medical school to show the rest of the medical world that it can be done.

There is no lack of money in the world as many believe. One only has to find out where it is and negotiate the terms of the agreement.

The essential behavior of every person is to earn or find the money to pay for the product or service they can't do without.

Why else would anyone pay $2,500 for a Super Bowl ticket when they could just as well watch it for free at home on their own TV set? Even the poorest of our population are magically able to find money for cigarettes and alcohol while living on the streets in rags and starving.

"The difference between an ordinary income and an extraordinary income is implementation."
-Bill Glazer

A closer look at funding and support opportunities

Without having the necessary information about the exact costs of creating a business education program for medical students, assumptions have to be made at this point.

With a list of the services and projects that would be necessary to *begin such a program*, the costs of accomplishing everything beginning to end in today's numbers can be made available. A reasonable estimate might be $2 million. Beginning with an amount about twice as much as the actual expense is predicted to prevent worries about cost overruns during the project.

The costs of maintaining such a program each year, including paying business experts for business education lectures, personnel to oversee the business education program, and constant updating all new content for the program materials and lectures would likely be at least $500,000 a year.

Once all the business study and lecture materials are created and then converted to digital formats of some kind for students, the annual maintenance costs would drop to half of the above maintenance costs—about $250,000.

Assuming these costs are within range of the real costs, then the break-even cost per medical student on an annual basis might be *about $1,600 per student*. It follows that the cost billed to students would be very reasonable indeed. However, as most cost estimates usually are half of the final real costs that are paid, it would still be a reasonable cost for each student to pay.

1. **Medical school alumni funds.**

Judging by the reported donations made by the members of my Perelman Medical School class of 1962, which seems to be one of the most responsive classes, even our class donations would not make a dent in the cost of funding business education for all medical students.

Adding up the total donated monies of all classes over many years, it might cover the costs of starting such a business education program, assuming the donations made were all earmarked for this cause.

2. **Other university alumni donations or anonymous donations from individuals or organizations.**

All monetary funds donated and applied to support the business education program from these three sources would require people with fundraising experience and expertise.

The most advantageous resource would probably be a very wealthy individuals interested in benefiting medical education of doctors. Most universities and medical schools have a current list of such donors already.

We know that Bill Gates, Warren Buffett, and Jon M. Huntsman, Sr. have a strong interest in improving healthcare by their personal philanthropy. Any billionaire who started in a garage behind his house (Bill Gates), started as a pinball machine repairman (Warren Buffett), or began by making egg cartons (Jon Huntsman, Sr.) are worth their salt—and are worth asking for help.

When such wealthy people also have a direct connection to the university, medical school, or business school, it gets a foot in the door.

All *masons* have been persistent and credible supporters of healthcare for more than a century in the US and Europe. They presently have over twelve children's hospitals they have built and maintain in the US and one in Mexico City that provide free care to children with many orthopedic and other medical illnesses. They also have a functioning healthcare system called "Rite Care."

As a member of this elite fraternal organization, I can assure you that they would be interested in helping fund the increased education (business education) of medical students should anyone choose to ask them and present the situation to them.

In case you haven't learned about the innovative efforts, influence, and accomplishments of the Masonic organizations in support of public education, government, healthcare and our society since it became a nation, I suggest you investigate their attributes and their potential for helping.

3. Companies that have always supported physicians, hospitals, and medical education.

Pharmaceutical companies have given out visual educational charts, patient education materials, and medication samples to doctors for patients for well over half a century as part of their marketing strategies, but these are also beneficial to our healthcare in many ways.

These companies are highly positioned to become even more helpful than they have been because there has always been mutual benefit for both parties.

It may be possible to persuade some of them to sponsor one or many of the medical students who are participating in the business education program. From a business point of view, that action would offer them a tremendous opportunity to have a doctor on the inside of the medical business world that would be subject to the laws of attraction and persuasion.

Physicians are biased towards these supportive companies in more ways than one. There was a time when nearly all physicians prescribed only brand-name drugs because their quality was guaranteed, rather than generic drugs whose quality varied considerably.

Physicians are direct instigators of hospitals to buy surgical instruments from reliable instrument manufacturers—another powerful connection. In other words, there are the human behavioral patterns that are well known to affect our actions that are not a very subtle part of our nature.

The Twelve Laws of Persuasion are used every day in marketing to other people and businesses all over the world.

In this situation, *the laws of connectivity, dissonance, expectation, involvement, obligation, verbal packaging, social validation, scarcity, esteem, contrast, balance, and association* produce an undercurrent of compliance often in a subconscious manner. They are a boon to the business of any pharmaceutical, medical supply, and medical instrument company.

All three of these may also be very good sources for sponsorship and donations to the business education cause.

Hospitals would also benefit from taking on sponsorship of medical students. Think about it: hospitals are now buying up financially failing medical practices and the doctors. The influence, business acumen and knowledge, and business skills of those doctors benefit any system they are part of.

These are smart people who are up to their tasks, in both marketing and business. They understand and are well informed about the concept of "strategy from the outside in," which is the most current and highly efficient marketing approach to customers. In their latest book, *"Strategy From the Outside In,"* George Day and Christine Moorman describe the most recent shift in marketing from the **Inside Out** process to the **Outside In** approach in detail.

What this book teaches all businesses is that starting out by researching what customers want and need today tells businesses what services and products they should be providing and offering customers and are the ones that are highly likely to become profitable for those companies.

Previously, the companies decided themselves what they believed customers needed and found their incomes dropping rapidly. Large companies like Dell Computer discovered that the "inside-out" format no longer works, and it has taken almost ten years to catch up to their competitors, Apple and HP. They caught up because they switched to the new marketing method.

All this means is that there is a *huge opportunity for medical schools* to tell those companies (marketing effort) what they want and need to obtain the reciprocal funds they would need for funding the business education of medical students.

"You can't see who's naked until the tide goes out."
-Warren Buffett

4. Organizations, countries, and businesses outside the USA:

Everyone knows that America has the greatest medical educational system in the world. Many other countries send students to us for business, medical, and other educational objectives.

Most foreign students are from families that have better than average financial resources. They send students here because they can afford the cost of the student's education. It seems reasonable that they can also afford the cost of a business education of their own country's medical students as well.

Hospitals, governments, and industries in other countries understand the value of an American education and are good candidates for becoming medical student sponsors or donors.

India in the past has required medical students who graduated from a foreign medical school to return to India for two years of practice before they are given a choice of where in the world they prefer to practice. To my knowledge, it's still true today.

India is one example that would likely be very interested in returning doctors who were educated in business as well as medicine. India is a rapidly advancing nation in world business. Their medical system is in bad need of repair to which returning business-educated doctors would be of enormous help.

5. Medical schools that share funding resources.

Certainly, if one medical school decides to start a business education program for their medical students, others will follow quickly. It's a very powerful recruiting strategy as well.

It's very possible that two or three of the top medical schools could work together to create a business education program for medical students and share the prestige and costs.

The arrangements for such a project would require a master negotiator with the passion of an elephant on a rampage and the process would take a lot less time to achieve than doing it all themselves.

It's doubtful that such an arrangement could be done simply because of the many conflicts involved between medical school and university competitors. However, for smaller and less affluent schools, it could be a smart business venture all around.

"You can't win by playing not to lose."
-Maxwell Maltz, MD

6. Medical students can bear the cost of an integrated medical-business education program.

Of all the possible financial arrangements made to pay for the coordinated medical-business education program for medical students, having the students pay the additional costs would seem to be a top-of-the-list approach for funding the program.

This approach might significantly increase student's educational debt, probably lose potential students as a result of the added costs, and might create an additional financial hardship later.

A quick uneducated guess about cost per student for the $500,000 cost for a medical school to maintain such a business education program per medical school class per year might run about $500,000 divided by 160 students per class is equal to $3,125 cost per student.

The probability that a young doctor with a formal business education under his belt would be able to pay off this part of the increased educational debt much quicker and with less worry is one-fifth the time it would take without the business knowledge. He or she would have the business marketing tools and knowledge to do it all right from the start of medical practice.

Banks would be more lenient on granting loans to new doctors when they know about their business education background and their more dependable capacity to pay off their educational debts.

Can you imagine today what happens when a new doctor, just out of residency training or internship, practically broke no job yet, loaded with educational debt, asks a banker for a loan to start a medical practice? His only asset and collateral is his word, educational background, and the fact that he gave the banker a hearty laugh to start his day.

7. Confiscating chunks of funds from other monies designated for other school purposes.

If our own government can get away with "robbing Peter to pay Paul" over and over again, medical schools can do the same, even legally. The difficulty is in convincing the decision-makers that formal business educations for all medical students will in the long run pay them back ten times over what they invest in the program. Smart people can figure that out to the dollar.

Everything is a risk, and business-educated people know that. Even educators know that. The fact that any new and much publicized educational program that's supposed to make miracles happen for physicians may fail, is a calculated risk that needs to be accepted. Marketing the program would be an excellent investment.

But one has to remember some realities that are present and shift the extent of the risk to minimal.

a. You are dealing with highly educated and motivated individuals unlikely to fail.

b. Every educator, physician, successful business person, knows that a *formal business education* of all professionals escalates profits, productivity, and financial stability of all businesses.

c. Educators know that medical students' minds are capable of handling the information and knowledge learned in the business program. This is supported by the fact that the brain recognizes, categorizes, and banks over an estimated two billion pieces of information brought to the brain through our five senses *every day*.

d. The education of and preparation for the success of every medical student is a primary mandate and is the responsibility of medical schools.

Whether medical school academics ignore it or not, a "formal business education" for all medical students is the only way of *ensuring* the capability for and the maximal success of accomplishments of every medical doctor.

e. It has been estimated by business experts that every doctor without a formal business education *leaves a million dollars on the table during their medical careers that they could have had* if they had adequate business knowledge to recognize it.

The person or administrative group of individuals that distribute the accumulation of donated funds for the purposes that are needed must carry the vision and passion for making the best decisions. These people make decisions based on priorities. As new projects are proposed, they are added to the list at the level of their agreed-upon importance to the institution.

Any project can be moved up or down on the list of priorities depending on its value and importance at that time. Logical reasoning would place the *business education of medical students at the top of the list* because of its intrinsic value to both students and the medical school.

Of course, there are many other factors that must be considered in those decisions. Social, political, and economic forces come to bear on every decision being made. However, when an essential project such as this is proposed, most of the influences affecting the decisions and priorities being made should be of secondary importance.

Compared with such things as the need and use of a new building on campus or the necessity for restructuring of the medical school staff and salaries, the creation of an *absolutely essential academic business education of medical students far surpasses any others.*

In addition, this focused business education project will be a longer, enduring, breathtaking, and transformational improvement in medical education for the benefit of all concerned. It just takes setting a goal and a deadline for its activation and its completion.

"Nobody can go back and start a new beginning, but anyone can start today and make a new ending."
-Anonymous

8. Crowdfunding and venture capital resources.

The rapidly expanding funding sources from both crowdfunding and venture capital are available for grabs. If you don't ask, then they don't offer nor go out searching for businesses that need money. In the past, medical practice has been well known to be a private business.

Private businesses employ over 60 percent of the nation's workforce. In the future, private businesses likely will employ a much higher percentage of workers based on what the country's economic future looks like.

For small businesses loans are much harder to obtain from various financial institutions. Thus, turning to these two resources for funding is the obvious choice for self-employed physicians and other small businesses at the present time. No doubt the government and politicians will soon put restrictions on these businesses. But until then, these friendly funding resources will continue their services.

Even though universities and medical schools are not private small businesses, they are in the eyes of these funding sources highly reliable candidates for paying back loans. Qualifications for funding are more personal in nature and much less restrictive than those of regulated funding sources.

9. Corporate funding possibilities.

For those marketing people who keep up with the rapid-fire pace of changes and trends in methods that corporations are now implementing, it's no surprise that corporations are looking at future threats to business and are already funding the educational resources that will protect their financial stability.

As reported in the *WSJ*, April 8, 2014, in an article titled, "Corporate Cash Alters University Curricula," the trend opens new opportunities for universities and medical schools to obtain funding for specific purposes. Undoubtedly, the wisdom of corporate minds have determined that they are no longer dealing with just another economic bubble that will burst and all will return to normal again.

What corporations (and medical schools should see) see in the future is the obvious ultimate calamity that *Harry Dent Jr., economics expert,* among others has been trying to warn our country and government about for several years: a total cataclysmic financial collapse of the USA and the world. Economic evidence of that is abundant, realistic, and credible.

When this will happen is anyone's guess. Our nation, including the majority of our nation's population and the government politicians voted into office by a misled ignorant public who are "Ruled by Pop Culture" (Andy Serwer, Managing Editor, *Fortune Magazine*) predictably will perpetuate the final happening. Millions of smart and informed people are preparing for it as well.

So until it actually happens, life continues as usual. But it doesn't mean that medical schools can't proceed and continue to advance efforts to improve the things they are capable of doing. That means establishing a necessary business education of all medical students and to secure the funding to do so from corporations, whose survival depends on the continued supply of intelligent business educated physicians.

The article noted above would certainly include the funding for medical schools for specific mutual benefit. An open "marketing mind" can see and understand the compatible specific corporation's security and survival needs relative to their absolute dependence on medical doctors, especially those who are formally business educated. Understandably, it will be a win-win partnership for everyone involved.

It's not difficult to understand that this funding approach may well be the most advantageous of all, and for many solid reasons.

Cost of various educational examples found in the *medical practice business* marketplace today.

The costs of various educational materials already available to physicians and medical students is another means of evaluating the extent of expense and funding of a business education that may be appropriate for starting a medical school business education for students.

If a medical school business education course was to be started at the lowest level of expense and yet provide enough current business information at an academic level so that every student would gain full benefit, then it should be presented as a digitally created sequence of academic business instruction materials and formats.

Such a program should be available in several formats because of the various means that students learn most efficiently. Some learn best by video presentations. Some learn faster and remember more by reading and by writing notes.

Others find that live lecture presentations are the easiest way for them to learn. Some prefer a mixture of these digital formats (well-advised best).

Digital formats such as CDs have some advantages. They are portable, and students can listen to them while driving or walking.

Digital formats such as DVDs have advantages that include video, hearing, text, and persuasive voice and image presentations. More information can be recorded on a DVD than a CD and therefore more information can be provided at one time or session.

Having the convenience of a computer, iPad, or other mobile device adds another dimension to learning opportunities. One can readily check references online on the spot without having to remind themselves to look them up later. The general familiarity of current medical students with all these materials and formats makes this path of teaching easier than most.

When these educational materials are downloaded to their own personal computers, the information can be viewed from almost anywhere on their mobile device or from another computer.

Printing manuals for students to keep or use permits them to have quick reference to the knowledge when other formats are not available-not that any medical student would ever think of reading the manual in the middle of a boring medical lecture.

With all CDs and DVDs learning is enhanced by also providing the same information in written materials and accompanying reports or manuals. Written materials are much easier to update when they are kept in a three-ring binder and a single page can be replaced (the same is true for updating office procedure manuals).

Updating a CD or DVD usually means one has to re-record the whole material. The same is true with video presentations. However, there are technological methods to update the materials without having to re-record them.

Real examples and costs of digital and other educational materials

The American College of Obstetricians and Gynecologists happens to be what I am most familiar with because as a Life Fellow of the college I receive catalogs about their educational products.

Here is a breakdown of costs of educational materials I have purchased from various resources.

1. **CD-ROMs/DVD-ROMs:**
   Costs range from $10 to $500, depending on the topic, importance, and rareness of the information.

2. **Resource toolkits:**
   (ex. medical education, teen care; medical education, partner violence) Cost: $40-$100

3. **Reference books:**
   Cost: $10-$150

4. **Medical practice guidelines:**
   Cost: $5-$300

5. **Periodicals:**
   Cost (online version): $450-$700
   Cost (print version): $800-$1,200

6. **Marketing merchandise:**
   (shirts, tumblers, scrubs, lab coats, iPad cases)
   Cost: $15-$50

7. **Business and legal resources:**
   Cost: $10-$100

8. **Prolog review and learning:**
   Costs: $100-$800 (for series modules)

9. **Miscellaneous resources:**
   (ICD-9-CM coding, ethics, FAQ coding)
   Costs: $50-$15

These can stimulate ideas, provide a price range for what any medical school can do, and give credibility to cost ranges when anyone needs a comparison for purchasing them.

Costs for live speakers/experts range from *free* to $10,000 per lecture in the business world depending on the topic and the credentials of the person.

Webinars and teleseminars are another teaching/learning model that can easily be recorded and sold to students. Most commercial business webinars and teleseminars online are free to customers, but are presented to attract buyers of their other related business products that tell the buyers how to use the information presented to them.

Medical education costs when I attended medical school from 1958-1962 were manageable when both my wife and I had outside jobs and no other financial support. But now medical school education costs have moved to levels where students are incapable of managing without outside jobs.

As a result, students are now being forced to incur debts so huge that decisions being made about their education have shifted almost totally towards the cost of medical education rather than the quality of medical education.

The seemingly irresolvable situation that is now dictating the necessity of immediate cash flow from their employment right after completion of their medical education and training to begin payment of the educational debts, has essentially erased their options for and anticipated early benefits of medical practice.

The two critical elements that can dramatically improve medical student's future choices are...

1. An *academic business education* while in medical school

2. Using the *knowledge, skills, and tools of an academic business education* that will enable them to pay off all educational debts in less than half the time it will take new doctors to pay them off

without a business education. Doctors who don't know how to maximize their income will essentially live the following fifteen to twenty years of their career in relative "professional poverty." Employed doctors don't have that choice.

Comments

I do not claim to be an expert in financing or fund raising. My suggestions to you are meant only to provide you with ideas about the factors I believe to be available today for consideration and that you are certainly much more familiar with.

My estimates about the cost of funding a business education of medical students may be far off from what may turn out to be much higher costs, as commonly happens. At least it's a starting place for those who are experts in this area of finances, and maybe even give them a bit of humorous delight.

The point behind this chapter is to scream out my mission to you so loudly that maybe it will reach the ears and minds of intelligent individuals that think as I do about the mandatory need for business education of medical students.

I have personal experience in the trenches of this war and have suffered from the lack of a formal business education as great numbers of other physicians have over the years.

I know that it is the one greatest advantage available to new doctors that will transform medical education overnight. I know that this may be one of the rare opportunities in the history of the medical profession when this addition to medical education will be possible, judging from the economic trends and egregious attacks on our profession happening today.

I know that private medical practice will be erased from the "book of medicine" if what I advise is not implemented as soon as possible. The fundamental disintegration of the healthcare industry and medical profession with it will continue to progress downwards because, as much as we think and hoped that our profession would sometime reach a point where our clout would be recognized and followed, is a myth of stellar proportion.

I know intuitively that today our war to remain in control of our professional destiny is lost, but there are other battles to be fought that, if we win, will maintain the integrity and legitimate position of the medical profession in our society with the respect that is deserved and earned.

I also believe that this war we are fighting cannot be won by defensive maneuvers that dominate our present battle strategy. I know that we must go on the offensive immediately. We can make the medical profession a much more formidable opponent if every graduating medical doctor is armed with the business weapons proven to keep medical businesses alive and well.

Someone has to change the outdated mindset of medical education pundits. Hopefully, someone who reads this book will have the position, power, expertise, and motivation to not only be able to visualize the importance of this project, but also the inspiration to make it happen.

CHAPTER 10

Political and Economic Dictates

"Why Let Political and Economic Wounds of Doctors Escalate the Demise of Our Profession, When the Prevention is as Simple as Providing a Business Education for Medical Students"

A broad pragmatic view of the financial distress resulting from the business ignorance of doctors in private medical practice should be enough for medical school academics to recognize the desperate need to implement a formal business education for all medical students.

WE HAVE NO means of going back and retroactively providing today's practicing physicians with a business education, but we can start today by removing the business handicap that medical students still face today.

Most respected intelligent minds who are staunch supporters of the medical profession and have a credible grasp of where our nation's healthcare is headed continue to focus *defensively* on how physicians can avoid being stuck indefinitely under the government restrictions and mandates that account for physicians' "professional poverty."

Others stop at analyzing the medical practice data, demographics, the best defensive strategies open to physicians, and the future takeover of medicine, but *offer no practical offensive opportunities for physicians.* Most offensive strategies are relegated to understanding business strategies. They exist and are used successfully by the commercial business entities, but never reach the level of being recognized as important or expedient to physicians as well as medical school education academics.

For example, all doctors and medical educators have understood for decades that physicians would be far better off if somehow they would have gained a full academic knowledge of business and marketing.

All physicians themselves have known for decades that they would be far better off in their careers and life if they had simply learned to use successful business strategies in the management of their medical office, financial affairs, and professional careers. Everybody knows those things. They aren't secrets. They're simply camouflaged by the intensive distractions and narrowed focus on curing medical problems.

Why then has business education of physicians been persistently disregarded by both physicians and medical education pundits?

There are no significant world-shaking recognized disadvantages that I can think of to having and maintaining cutting-edge business proficiency. Such proficiency requires time, ongoing updating of business education, and self-discipline. All these specific requirements are the same as those that all physicians are already doing in their practice of medicine.

Let me summarize for you the reasons for physicians disregarding this essential component (business education) of the private practice of medicine that I hear all the time, like...

1. It's not convenient.
2. It's not mandatory.
3. It's not "time invested" that will help me much.
4. It costs me money.
5. It wastes my time.
6. It would overwhelm me to do that.

I'm sure there must be over fifty more responses that could be added to this list. But with a little "thought archeology," one can see the underlying causes so well hidden.

Clearly, there are a few underlying and understandable emotional factors that commonly overcome our logic and self-determination.

1. **Fear**: Such fears as going further into educational debt, spending time with business things when I should be seeing medical patients and earning income, worrying about whether I can learn all these business things or even want to, fear that these business things would not work in my kind of practice and whether I could afford to do them, fear about failing in medical practice, and others.

2. **Income insecurity**: A close connection to fear. This one monumental issue stands alone as the single trigger for jump-starting the business education revolution in the medical education of doctors. This factor is responsible for the vast number of reasons for physicians quitting, or being forced out of medicine prematurely.

   A physician's satisfaction with and passion for the practice of medicine is dependent almost entirely on the fulfillment of his or her early perceived and believed expectations that a career in medical practice offered. When the real truth about never being able to reach those expectations surfaces, the excitement of practicing medicine transforms into the hopeless attitudes we see so widespread among doctors in private practice today.

   If you do a survey of long-employed physicians, you will most certainly find that those same hopeless attitudes have been present for decades before today and for the same reasons.

   Don't be enticed to dive into the employment pond by the seemingly good incomes ($200,000-$400,000 on average) in nine-to -five day-jobs that *employed physicians* now take home.

   When you review the *SK&A (A Cegedim Company)* (*www.skainfo.com*) listings of good salaries (*See Appendix 4, page 325-330*) being paid to various categories of employed physicians, don't feel that you are missing the big salary bonanza. Because things will change very soon under the increasing Obamacare restrictions you may end up in a much better income situation.

   Those salaries being paid today will surely be greatly reduced as soon as private medical practice is eliminated. Read more about SK&A (*Appendix 3, page 323-324*).

   If you think that government-controlled/restricted medical practice and the full impact of forced reduction of medical care costs that will eventually worsen, don't be surprised when HMO employers start firing doctors and lowering their salaries to meet the cost control measures forced on them as well.

These salaried and well-paid employed doctors today will likely soon be earning the same salaries that the average private doctors are earning today.

In addition, if you are an employed physician and don't meet the "patient visit" quotas required and are let go, it will be very difficult to find another employed physician position to apply for. Even today, physicians have a difficult time finding medical jobs that are *satisfactory* to them.

Now imagine the leverage you would have if you had an academic business education under your belt. You likely would be at the head of the line for jobs and at a better salary. A formal business education has more prestige and power than you think.

3. **Skepticism mindset:** This is probably the most destructive emotion for most doctors. Business experts have proven this over and over again. Physicians refuse to even talk face to face with a business expert anymore, to their detriment. What is so interesting about this fact is that almost all other professional medical care providers are very open minded about learning efficient, profitable, and productive business strategies.

   Why such a difference? Could it be arrogance? Likely it's because physicians were never even told that a business education would enhance their career and income thirty-fold.

As I look at this educational *business deficiency* in medical school education, it shocks and saddens me that this deficiency is tolerated among the medical profession academics and also rejected as a necessity by the majority of physicians practicing today.

First, I believe that the disbelief about the usefulness and value of a business education springs from the basic ignorance among physicians about what business and marketing does for a medical practice. Would you pay any attention to a person trying to sell you a deep-sea diving suit if you were never exposed to what it was good for?

Second, I believe that other physicians who reject the necessity for a business education, even when they see the advantage of it for themselves, is rooted in the ignorant and mythical view about not needing a business education to run a medical business. The implied belief that it is useless is fed subliminally (never mentioned) to them as medical students by uninformed faculty (business-wise).

After all, the faculty likely has become so accustomed to a salary that they would have no need or desire to "infect" medical students with real business principles, especially when they don't even know themselves.

Some pseudo-philosophical thoughts about medical school education and the status of physicians in our culture

Last night I stumbled on to a TV program about physicians. A physician oncologist named Otis Brawley, MD, had written a book entitled *"How Do We Harm: A Doctor Breaks Ranks about Being Sick in America."*

His theme was a long dissertation about the book about how physicians have been practicing medicine over many decades by over-treating and undertreating patients and how that has harmed patients.

He gave many examples of how these things happen, from too many C-sections and hysterectomies to treatments of breast cancer starting with Halstead's radical mastectomies continued into the 1980s.

Along with all of his statistics about survival rates and medical literature studies about effectiveness of treatments of various medical problems came the notion that physicians, although intending to treat patients properly, get carried away with treatments that are unnecessary or performed because they were misled by drug companies and medical literature.

If I had not been a physician listening to him, I would have been persuaded that most doctors are stretching the boundaries of good practices in healthcare and are moving much farther away from evidence based medical practice—which is harming patients.

He was right! But he completely ignored the reasons physicians are being forced into these private practice survival situations. That issue demands a transparent discussion about the realities of stretching private medical practice survival activities verses the publicly acceptable and seemingly tolerable corruption permeating every institution in our nation, and I dare say, the world.

> *Shall we continue to have the advantage of healthcare provided by private medical practice of independently thinking doctors?*
>
> *Or shall we accept all healthcare provided only by physicians that are tightly controlled by medical practice restrictions which result in limitations on their skills and medical knowledge?*

YOU KNOW WHAT I MEAN—physicians who are essentially held hostage by controlling employers who pay their salaries while bent on tight controls of healthcare costs.

Physicians who don't meet the established quotas of patients seen per day and treated or become resistant in any manner to the established system are quickly terminated (based on subjective decisions made without appeal process). And you also know that there is a long waiting list of doctors eager to take his or her place in the system.

What I objected to was that Dr. Brawley neglected to present many of the realities of the private practice of medicine and medical treatments. It's always the same context of stories and presentations, examples and explanations, which one expects to hear from "lecturing physicians" who spend their whole practice life as an employee, either on government payroll or on that of other entities.

They have no real concern about their own honesty of providing opposing evidence or circumstances about what happens to physicians in private medical practice. Therefore, they are able to sway the listening audience the majority of the time to their way of thinking and mislead patients and the public about their personal stand on a topic.

For example, the problem of overuse of C-section deliveries is worsening. He never mentioned the enormous risk present in obstetrical practice associated with malpractice risks, lawsuits, and their direct effects on doctor's medical decisions about delivering babies.

Another example is that new medications that cost twenty times as much per dose as older medications that are just as effective are being prescribed. He never mentioned that problem private practice doctors have in trying to make patients believe that a C-section is *more risky* than vaginal delivery or that the old cheap drug is just as effective as the new one when patients come into the office demanding the treatment or drugs they want. Patient demands cost millions of dollars and altered my medical practice approach permanently.

To keep patients in their medical practice and to keep enough patients to earn enough so they can pay the practice overhead and have enough net income to live a professional lifestyle, doctors either cater to patients demands or close their practice; this is a well-known fact.

These are a few of the private practice problems and borderline ethics physicians face to remain solvent in practice and that aren't publicized or talked much about:

1. If doctors refuse to follow patient demands, they will likely lose those patients. But doctors are obligated to explain why. That rarely prevents a patient from going elsewhere. Employed doctors have no problem with a patient's reaction because they get paid regardless of their stand on questionable practice activities.

2. When doctors spend 20 percent of their time on medical paperwork and 20 percent of their time on keeping up with the current medical literature, there isn't much time left to see and treat medical patients and it compromises their family life every day.

   I knew an internal medicine doctor who claimed that his vast current medical knowledge was the result of reading medical literature four hours every day after he got home from the office. I always wanted to ask him how his family life was doing, but never did.

3. The public is totally ignorant of the problems doctors really have in medical practice and just assume erroneously that they are all rich or well paid.

I've gone through this discussion for one essential reason: to give you another reason why providing a business education for medical students has even more importance today. If the medical academic world gives a twit about doing something about the highly stressful private medical practice lives of physicians they graduate—about twenty thousand a year from all medical schools in the nation, then let them show it.

Wouldn't you think that there are likely hundreds of smart medical education academics in our nation that should be ashamed of their complete disregard for making the necessary improvements (a business education) of medical student education and to give medical students a reliable chance of having a satisfying medical practice career? Most private practice physicians don't have that today!

What must be done by the medical profession to properly serve their members?

If medical practice is seriously considered a *legal business entity*, then it requires the business and marketing knowledge of the owner to plan, create, maintain, protect, upgrade, and grow that medical business for it to have any reasonable possibility for success or survival.

If medical practice *does survive* somehow *without* the business requirements necessary for any reasonable amount of business income and success, it will happen only because physicians have other sources of income outside medical practice. And that factor should become a profound objective for physicians who disregard a business education.

Physicians have never been expected to provide medical care for free. There was a time when money was not the primary driver for practicing medicine. Today it is.

It's a basic economic reality. When millions of customers are knocking down your doors to buy your services, there is no need to advertise or for marketing your medical practice services.

Simple and logical maneuvers in the past like those above have coincidentally permitted survival of medical practices without a practicing physician knowing anything about running a medical business.

There are no more manipulations left to try to counter the extreme changes that have happened in our society and economy and that permit a medical practice to survive today without the physician having a supreme knowledge of business strategies and tools.

Cultural, societal, political, and economic changes have changed everything regarding healthcare and the practice of medicine. These combined changes and factors require doctors to have business knowledge as well as a medical knowledge to survive in private medical practice.

First, it's time for the medical profession to go outside the profession and *promote itself far and wide*, because the virtues and dignity of the profession have been slowly chipped away by medical malpractice attorneys, politicians, and the media to the point that the medical profession in the eyes of the public has become so weak, even dangerous, that it seems mid-level providers are considered more dependable and trustworthy than physicians.

What is almost completely lacking is a *widespread ongoing direct mail campaign* promoting the following...

1. The importance and advantages of fee-for-service healthcare.

2. The importance and special advantages of private medical doctors and their practices that can't be found at managed care facilities.

3. The advantages and benefits to patients being cared for by private medical doctors. Often we see in the media information about the benefits of healthcare by managed care doctors and facilities.

So far, I haven't received one single piece of direct mail advocating ways to save private medical practice and prevent the attrition of doctors. Nor have I seen or read articles, editorials, or information in the media over the last couple years, with few exceptions, about how caring and competent most private practice doctors truly are.

It's not to say that behind closed doors within the medical profession hierarchy such discussions haven't been undertaken many times.

The public seems to be relying on the media, politicians, and trends of the U.S. Congress to explain what's happening today to the practice of medicine, and it is rarely about the real story about private medical practice. We hear lots of opinions and editorials about changes in healthcare and the effects of those changes, but not about the effects on those who deliver the healthcare: *professional medical care providers.*

Anyone who has read the opinion of Scott W. Atlas, MD (*WSJ May 1, 2014*), senior fellow at Stanford University Hoover Institute, about the coming *two-tier health system*, has the clearest view of the future of healthcare as well as the increasing challenges physicians will be facing just to remain in medical practice in the very near future. He's correct, I believe.

The public needs to *hear directly from physicians, medical organizations, and medical schools* as well as all the associated medical institutions that support the medical profession faithfully about the quality, competence, and trustworthiness of doctors today.

The positive impact comes from testimonials, unsolicited reports, peer reviewed medical journals, medical journalists who understand the battle going on, and patients who have had good experiences in their healthcare that need to be publicized far more often than they are today.

The media is quite inspired to publish the errors doctors make, the stories about their legal problems, and the patient injuries caused by certain surgical procedures and drug reactions.

The AMA has spent millions of dollars lobbying congress regarding medical care delivery and has had very little ROI with that effort. Once in a while they report something in the newspapers that they have done. The last one was a ten-line bit in the *WSJ* about an effort to push for renovating medical school education—and nothing since; no follow up.

Like this one-shot message, never repeated or followed-up with results and progress, most are a single issue or report that no one follows up on. I'll tell you one thing: Whoever is in charge of their marketing likely doesn't understand marketing principles. The same is true for most medical organizations who don't know what they don't know about marketing.

If medical pundits in the hierarchy of the medical profession think that publishing all the wonderful accomplishments of physicians and medical researchers only in medical journals really gets out to the public, medical patients, and other collaborating elements of the medical profession, it doesn't.

Why is it that most all of the great things happening in healthcare and the medical profession either remain silent within the profession or require some media medical reporter to seek out those impressive accomplishments and inform the public?

I think that relying on the liberal press to filter through those in-profession publications and to report on them while including their own biases as well as that of the editors of the paper often backfires.

Why is it that the medical profession doesn't have its own marketing department doing those positive promotions of the medical profession?

Medicine is really big business and should be promoting itself if for no other reason than to maintain its "brand", purpose, services, uniqueness, values, and integrity. You will see it sometimes coming from doctor's offices, but nothing much from the great centers of the medical profession.

Paid medical newsletters published by big medical centers is nothing more than a wart on marketing's finger and misses the concept of promotion.

It's good business to keep those ideals always in the public eye. Otherwise all the public hears and sees is the dark side of the profession.

The medical profession needs a *positive spin* on our position in our society and an *offensive strategy* to help dissipate the hopelessness doctors feel today.

Medical Economics (April 10, 2014) reported that physicians contribute ten million jobs and $1.6 trillion to the economy according to AMA reports.

Who cares? Only the readers of that magazine, who are usually health care professionals, get that message, not the regular voting citizens who get that kind of mail in their mailbox and rarely pay attention to media reports.

Over 52 percent of physicians (2012 survey by Merritt-Hawkins for the Physician Foundation) have already dumped their Medicare and

Medicaid patients or intend to. Add to that the rise of those patients from 107 million to 135 million in the next five years and we have to wonder who will be seeing those patients.

If all upcoming graduating physicians were formally business educated, it's likely there would be many more physicians available to treat them, who otherwise would not be able to earn enough to afford to keep their medical practice open. Nobody reports about that. All the public hears is that doctors are complaining about reduced fees, not the real story.

When physicians reach the point when there are only two choices for practicing medicine—concierge practice or practice as an employee—the ranks of concierge physicians will predictably skyrocket in numbers. The cash-only method of practice will be available only to patients with money or have expensive private health insurance coverage.

Dr. Atlas also points out that since the great majority of the top medical doctors and best hospitals in the nation will remain outside of Obamacare (ACA), all patients with Obamacare will be managed by a population of doctors and hospitals willing to exist on the borders of bankruptcy. It means that the quality of healthcare will be reduced.

Have you ever seen *that message* widely spread by the media to the majority of the population?

Has our population been informed about what's happening in Europe, all of whom have a government-run health care system? There must be a lot of patient dissatisfaction there when you know that two-thirds of British citizens earning over $78,000 a year, for example, purchase private health insurance and fifty thousand British citizens travel outside the country annually to obtain healthcare.

Is our public blind to the number of Canadian patients who move to the USA for healthcare or Canadian doctors who move to the USA to practice medicine?

There is abundant evidence and proof that our own physicians are desperate to improve their incomes and medical practice competence. At the same time it seems there is ample evidence that if physicians don't earn enough money to meet their expectations they will leave the profession and physician attrition will persist.

The *offensive way* to prevent that is to educate all physicians in business principles and strategies that will enable them to earn what they need by using the tools of business, which they don't have now.

The developing new look at medical business education possibilities.

In chapter 8 of this book, I describe some options as to how a formal business education could be efficiently provided to medical students. That discussion was based on how a formal business education can be provided to medical students in the least expensive and efficient manner. Now I want to expand on that view to take in the newer alternatives being experimented with today within the global and international view.

Several of the most prestigious business schools, such as the University of Pennsylvania's Wharton School of Business (most aggressive), Virginia's Darden School of Business, and Harvard Business School, have made some remarkable steps into developing online business education courses, some free and some paid. Other business schools are slow to take the bait.

Might that move to put business education online have happened because of the fact that most students who need and want that education won't take the time to get it otherwise, nor spend the serious money to do it on-campus? Doctors and medical students are no different.

The Wharton Business School, while taking this challenge and concept seriously, has already begun the process of planning massive open online courses to reach millions of students desiring business education. Their goal is to provide basic business skills to those who are unable to pay full tuition for such education.

The business courses are free to take, and no credits are given towards a business school degree. It's interesting that Wharton's thought is to teach these courses to educate students about what business knowledge will do to improve their lives in any business or career and how it works to accomplish that. By learning the basics, a student then is able to see the importance of a complete business education is to their career—a formidable strategy.

This is what I preached back in chapter 8 when I explained that medical students have no idea how important a formal business education is because no one has taken the time to tell them the facts. It's also the reason doctors today refuse to get a formal business education later: because they have never understood the importance and advantages it has for them.

Whoever made the decision to do this at Wharton certainly understands the basic marketing strategy and remarkable advantages of "being the first" in most any commercial enterprise. Medical schools should start thinking seriously about moving themselves into *first position* to provide a formal business education of all medical students.

Wharton's courses run $20,000-$50,000 to create depending on the professor's involvement in the production and editing of the course. The University of Pennsylvania gets a small cut of any profits.

Wharton's online business courses are made available through Coursera, Inc. and are different from the real business school curriculum, which involves much more intensive materials, research, and business strategies. Their plan is to eventually provide the majority of the MBA content online, but not for free.

It's not difficult to implement at least parts of such a business education program into the medical education curriculum today.

New focus for business schools

Most business school students today are gunning for banking, consulting, and technology jobs. (*WSJ-May 1, 2014, article by Melissa Korn about MBAs*) The global financial crisis is being blamed for a lack of a world view about business and the lack of adequate business education of business decision makers along those lines.

Some business scholars are pushing for decisions being made based on an international business background in theory, history, and philosophy related to economics in the world. The idea is to solve a problem with a world view and not based on local circumstances and ideas.

Students are becoming more aware of the need for a better understanding of marketing and business dynamics in addition to the entrepreneurial approach to finding a way to solve any business problem.

This seems to indicate that there is a significant deficiency in the core of business education and needs to be upgraded—the same that presently exists in the medical school education system.

What I believe to be the absolutely essential dynamic that's necessary to effectively teach a formal business education to medical students.

The one fallible aspect of teaching is to be able to make a direct and lasting connection between learning and the *real experiences of living the lesson.*

In the case of medical students or future physicians yet in college, the unique problem facing educators is that of leading the minds of those individuals into the world of business while implanting an intense desire to continue to learn and use their business knowledge to magnify their unique career choices.

In one way or another, all income in life has its origin from some form of business entity.

It's a preparation process for students to develop their own mental mechanism for connecting and adapting business principles to most everything they do in life. That business passion of students should be initiated while in college premed and preferably long before then.

However, in medical school education, to this day there has been no mind preparation or development of a passion for learning about business. Consequently, if one is to create a business passion and also teach students how to apply business strategies and tactics to their career of medical practice at the same time, a unique method of teaching them about business is required.

The two factors that demand a different approach than is usual for learning to apply business principles to the business of medical practice are that medical students will be learning and digesting two different categories of education, business and medical, at the same time. Dual educations have been running in higher education since I was a medical student: our school offered a combined PhD and MD program at the time.

The second factor is that without any prior academic business preparation, as is the case of nearly all starting medical students; students must promptly recognize the necessity for and importance of a continuing interaction between business and medical practice for the duration of their medical careers.

There are many avenues of approach to enable such a dual education. It's not a matter of a student's brain power or IQ. It's not a matter of having enough time to get it done. It's not a matter of it being too expensive to provide to students. It's not a matter of whether business or medical education is the most important to students.

It is a matter of developing the entrepreneurial spirit lying dormant in every medical student who has ever graduated from medical school. You may have noticed that over the last five years at least, an increasing number of universities and colleges are adding courses in "Entrepreneurship." Awakening the eyes and ears of educators is a dramatic turnaround for higher education that has discovered this dormant muscle in the brain.

Medical students already have the desire and passion for learning. It seems to reach its maximum intensity ever on the first day of medical school. Am I right?

The next step is to connect business and medical practice in the minds of students in such a way that it is easy to understand and bring together in a very realistic and practical manner. That's the key to the whole process in a nutshell.

One means of connecting business directly to medical practice is by presenting the two experiences live. By using real live examples of business solutions to medical practice problems that every private practice physician is facing today, it strikes the core of every student's expectations from his or her medical career.

The ultimate and most effective means of impacting the minds of medical students about the necessity of obtaining business knowledge is to require them to spend time with a private practicing doctor.

Live practicing doctors standing in front of the class talking about these issues does make a lasting and profound impact.

Many medical schools offer electives to students. Electives for further in-depth studies about business would be very helpful.

Preceptorships, with actively practicing doctors in the local area, are even more beneficial. Imagine following a good doctor around for six or eight-weeks, morning to night, in his or her private practice. Is there any better way to see the truth about needing a business education?

Visualize being allowed to look at actual finances and management processes while noting the deficiencies and problems involved in those areas of practice.

Think about those hundreds of questions you could ask that doctor and have the privilege of his blunt and honest answers.

Another important means of connecting business to medical practice is to arrange to have well-known business experts give lectures to medical school students, but provide consultation services to doctors in practice. This opens up a whole new area of information about doctors and medical practices that most doctors would never admit themselves.

Doctors are very touchy about confessing to blunders, stupid decisions they've made, and other facts that make them appear dumb or stupid. We all are guilty of those things, but we learn a lesson each and every time. It means that we all continue to learn throughout our careers and our lives. Since we are always learning, keep updating ourselves on business strategies and medical issues, it's not far out of the way to improve on it.

There are no limitations to what the brain can remember and store in our memory banks (*see image on page 131)*. Therefore, the issue of the importance of a formal business education and the implementation of such a curriculum into the present medical school education curriculum should be neither difficult nor delayed one more day.

Has any college ever tried this unique idea? Or even seriously considered it?

Idea: A combined "*college education*" that would include a formal business education and college degrees for both.

How about creating a four year BS + MBA curriculum, even a BS + MBA program for premeds?

It's not as crazy as it may sound and I'm certainly not the first one to look at such an opportunity. The process might create a relevant construct for colleges for being more than institutions that simply enable students to get a job.

The creation of such combined programs is not new to the education process. Combined programs and degrees just haven't been adapted to the new goals of college education using any widely accepted promotional advantages.

Some colleges and universities have already taken the hint by creating courses in entrepreneurship. The thinking behind that curriculum certainly is to develop the creativity, independent thinking, self-discipline, and decision making competence to solve any and all problems in business in particular.

An even more important factor is that the entrepreneurship process connects directly with creating businesses and careers. The *one thing that's missing*, and hopefully will soon be added, is learning how to create and run a business efficiently and profitably by using business principles and marketing strategies that create successful businesses.

Combined degrees should be a four-year+ education or year-round education process.

A combined college degree process could easily be used to prepare premed students well enough for medical school and professional medical careers. The combined degree program (BS + MBA + premed) would be an incredible advantage in many ways to both the university and the premed class.

The result for premed students would give them a significant leg up for acceptance to medical schools, job positions after graduation, changing careers, and lifelong knowledge about business anywhere they end up.

Universities who do this would have a huge marketing advantage, academic advantage for recruiting the best students, and much greater prestige among the post-graduate education and professional schools.

Just the fact that such dual programs would be already adding business knowledge to graduating students that in most all cases will not later ever get such an important education, at least in the case of physicians in their medical training and careers.

Like Martin Luther King said, *"I have a dream."* Don't we all?

The impact goes far beyond just wounding physicians.

This crippling lack of a formal business education also infects the professional lives of many of the other healthcare providers and professionals who own a healthcare business or manage one.

Take dentists for example. Dentists are just as injured by the *anti-business conspiracy* (did I just say that?) and predestined for financial failure for the same reasons as physicians.

However, dentists are rapidly becoming smart enough to take the time to find and learn from professional business educators like Dan S. Kennedy, among others. Business experts are more than excited and proud to help medical providers like dentists and chiropractors learn to become smart business people. Unfortunately, it's something that physicians have a hard time grasping and taking advantage of.

I've read recently that law schools (*WSJ June 30, 2014, by Jacob Gershman*), have introduced innovative courses to draw new students because of sharply falling enrollment. Yale Law School offers a crash course in Piketty-mania (which focuses on the views of French economist Thomas Piketty). Georgetown University Law School offers a seminar in regulation of "autonomous (robots) agents." Pepperdine University Law School offers videogames for helping students who are locked into procrastination escape that restrictive behavior.

The reason I mention this is because law schools don't teach their students about how to run their law practice businesses. Instead, they seem to want to provide complete distractions that are more contemporary or quirky. Can entertainment also teach us?

What one can draw from this is that creating entertainment for law students is more important to educational law scholars than providing a sound business education for lawyers. Ultimately, this leads to financial failure of solo law practices the same as physicians face in their practices. It also pushes law students into employment positions the same as is happening to physicians.

This situation may have something to do with the rapidly increasing segment of the legal profession who prey on physicians and healthcare industries by using medical malpractice litigation. Such medical malpractice litigation has become a formidable income producer for attorneys, and will continue to be a cash cow for attorneys.

Admittedly, medicine is an extremely complicated profession that functions in an environment of human diagnosis and treatment of healthcare problems, about which much is still unknown. Mistakes, injuries to patients, complications, and poor treatment results are expected and are fertile territory for lawsuits and income for attorneys.

If attorneys had an academic business education while in law school instead of superfluous courses (as also seen in medical schools), maybe the legal profession would have the capacity to financially do well without using the medical profession as their lucrative resource.

So what is going on today among a variety of professionals during their education is a complete disregard of a business education they need to survive, even to reach their maximal level of skills and knowledge. Skills and knowledge can only be attained when professionals are business knowledgeable enough to earn the income they need to get them.

The fact that the Internet, digital innovations, and online education now offer unlimited numbers of formats for students to learn from and educators to provide them with allows any school to provide a business education to students easily and consistently. Does anybody see a trend here to follow?

The new communication formats now enable every school to provide students with a formal academic business education and do it in a manner that students today are already well attuned to and are using.

CHAPTER 11

The Case Review

"Conclusions that Validate the Critical Value and Benefits of Including an Academic Business Education within the Medical School Education Curriculum"

About 172 medical schools in the USA have the responsibility and capability to provide a formal business education during the students' medical education. The perpetuating professional advantages for both young doctors, the medical school itself, the integrity of the medical profession, and the healthcare of our nation is no less than paramount to a medical history making endeavor.

IF THE TRUE purpose and objective of academic medical scholars is to *fully prepare* medical students with the knowledge, experience, and training necessary for the highest quality of expertise in the delivery of healthcare to patients, then it logically and sensibly obligates the decision to include an academic business education to comply with that goal.

Understandably, the continuing medical education, continued improvement of medical skills, and the continued ability of a doctor to afford to comply with these professional requirements *necessitates earning enough income* to be able to do so. Earning enough income for those necessities requires an academic business education.

When any physician lacks adequate income from their medical practice to do so, it seriously restricts their capacity and opportunities to maintain their skills and knowledge as well as their ability to increase them.

This factor of adequate income in private medical practice is restricted by the ever-increasing governmental fee restrictions, compliance with government laws and mandates, and migration of available medical patients to managed care facilities.

The only reasonable alternatives for physicians to increase their incomes to a satisfactory level are to work harder and face burnout, frustration, and failure. The desirable and effective means to know how to market and manage the business of their practices is to increase the flow of new patients in significant numbers and to retain older patients. The question is how to do that.

Most physicians don't own outside businesses or have outside sources of income, although these resources are rapidly becoming requirements for private medical practice survival.

To streamline their medical practice business (make it efficient) they need a formal business education to know how to do it and to make it effective. Rarely can you find a medical doctor today who truly knows how it's done profitably and effectively.

To continue and to grow a medical practice, a physician in today's world needs to know the marketing side of medical business thoroughly.

Since an academic business education includes marketing education, a physician with these tools has the capability of earning as much money as he or she needs to reach all their goals and pay for all their financial obligations to their family.

Problems employed physicians will have and can actually use a business education to resolve.

As I have discussed before in this document, employed physicians have been locked into contracts where salaries are fixed, and all business activities are handled by the owner or facility management group (remember the term "sacrificial lamb?").

With the repeated political efforts, now in 2014, to reduce healthcare costs, it's quite possible that employed physician's salaries will be reduced annually with no means of increasing their medical income under the contract requirements (which often forbid contract doctors from participating in or working for any outside business for income as a second job).

Physicians employed by hospitals are in a particularly vulnerable situation. Government control and actual influence on how hospitals function has already become a massive attack on the ability of hospitals to economically survive. So, which employees do they fire first? Probably the highest paid ones; like doctors and administrative nurses.

When employed some physicians discover their personal incompatibility with being employed. Therefore, they usually enter private practice in order to be their own boss. Here's another group of doctors who will also benefit tremendously from a business education.

It has been shown that of the 50 percent of graduating medical students, who now are seeking employed positions, about 12-15 percent will leave their employed position in a few years for various reasons.

After my personal experience of being an employed physician for about fourteen years of my medical career (military, Kaiser, hospital), I can righteously say that the best doctors are the ones who leave employed positions. My belief stems from what those physicians related to me personally as their reasons to leave their employment.

This's why an academic business education should be provided for every medical student during medical school.

A physician's future is unpredictable. That's because at the time of their decision-making, no graduating medical student knows what their practice circumstances will be later on—and it will be too late to get a business education for most doctors; they won't get it later for sure.

The primary reasons and undeniable factors that validate the proposal that medical students must have (not simply *think* it's a good idea) an academic business education:

1. *A medical practice is a real business* and must be managed as a real business to be maximally successful. It can't be done without a formal business education.

2. A physician is not capable of running a medical practice business at its maximum efficiency or profitably without a significant business education.

3. A medical practice business must adhere to the *same standards* required for the optimal success of any business.

4. When a medical practice is managed by a doctor with essentially no prior business knowledge and education, the practice is most often doomed to failure, at least to some degree below the doctor's actual capability.

5. Medical schools, who graduate students ignorant of their responsibilities for running the business that enables them to earn money from their medical practice, predestines every student to financial failure of their medical practice.

6. The responsibility of medical schools to provide a business education of medical students is validated by *the inevitable behavior of doctors* to avoid their own responsibility to obtain a business education on their own.

   Therefore, over 98 percent of doctors will choose to live with a poorly functional and inefficient medical practice because they have not learned how critical their business education is to their own survival and career.

7. The usual requirements for a Masters in Business Administration do not meet the *practical needs* of practicing doctors for many reasons. A business education must be *closely aligned to medical practice functions*, as it would be if provided to medical students.

   The reason for this is that doctors are disciplined to be focused 98 percent on medical practice and only secondarily and involuntarily on the practice business. The same is true for all professional medical care providers, such as dentists.

   You might have noticed the recent proliferation of media information concerning the increased effectiveness of education when students perform internships in businesses they intend to prepare for.

8. *A university or college business school education is not geared to the medical profession practice business*, but supplies the basics for

running any business profitably. It's just not good enough or specific enough for doctors to grasp well enough!

In this situation and for it to be most advantageous to physicians, basic business education must be seen and believed by medical students/physicians in a new and applicable light.

The business side of medical practice must be seen and acknowledged by medical educators and doctors (medical students as well) to be *equally as important to their maximal productivity and accomplishment* in their careers. Today the medical knowledge and skills they attain in their education is erroneously assumed to be the only pillars of their success.

Changing this unfortunate mindset requires time and enlightening instruction that offers physicians a viable means of magnifying their potential without seeding their minds with demands and threats. The **mistake** is to perpetuate the idea that business education should be *accomplished as a separate entity* from medical education.

Hopefully, this stands as a strong convincing and authoritative reasoning for providing a business and marketing education during the four-year medical student pursuit of medical education.

Wouldn't it be a fantastic experience for any medical school to witness the extraordinary accomplishments of all physicians who have graduated with an academic business-medical education that far exceed all expectations of the academic medical community? **It is** a reality.

Being a new revolutionary education model for medical/business education is one thing, but to be the one single dynamic improvement in healthcare that will drag physicians out of the quicksand of financial failure (a major disincentive facing most doctors in private practice of medicine today) is another.

While we all are sadly very aware of the gradual demise of private medical practice in our nation. And there doesn't seem to be any means of saving it today—is a terrible shame to live with.

The fact that we have obviously been forced to accept this impending fate without effectively battling back against the forces of government, politics, and turncoat influences that are greasing the slide we are now on indicates to me something is lacking that is very obvious to those with intelligent minds.

It seems that we are so consciously fixed on trying to reduce the threats against private practice from outside entities that we have forgotten how to fall back and fortify ourselves with while our reinforcements arrive.

Furthermore, it doesn't mean that there aren't other ways to fight back. Every physician with an advanced medical/business education is a warrior against suppression of medical practice freedom. A physician with these weapons has the ability to compete at the level of the economic playing field that our enemy has chosen for their intrusions.

Consequently, with this hybrid education process in play, physicians are ultimately prepared to chip away at the enemy's armor from a position of power, numbers, and winning strategies.

It may not seem on the surface to be effective enough to do much good. But over time, the concept has definite probability. What else do we have to help us survive?

No one expected David to slay Goliath, right?

9. *The nature of the medical profession is to compete with itself* and thus contributes to the disintegration of the medical profession as we have known it. Let me explain that.

   There are three distinct and "separate thinking" elements that divide the medical profession. These separate segments have completely different beliefs about what the ultimate goal of the profession should be, how to get there, and who should be the leaders and survivors.

The three elements or segments are:

a. Private-practice physicians

b. Physicians captured and bonded to employment lives

c. Physicians working within the academic and administrative areas of the medical profession

Superficially, the three elements function as one mind with many objectives. Deeper investigation shows that these three elements function independently and that each has a different single primary objective. This is well illustrated by the incompatible interaction and beliefs between the academic and private practice worlds.

Mindset factors that disconnect them.

Ask any medical doctor working in the academic world of teaching hospitals, medical schools, medical research, or even moderately interactive with these professional areas to explain to you in any significant detail the major problems facing private practice doctors today.

You will rapidly recognize the indifference being extruded primarily from among the academics, but also to a lesser degree from the others in this group. The indifference is far greater on the academic doctor's side and decidedly less on the private practice doctor's side.

The factors and beliefs on both sides result from (but rarely are discussed) their medical practice environment and positioning.

1. The common universal belief that will never be admitted "I practice in an area of medicine that is much more beneficial to patients than yours."

2. Doctors in academic medical teaching roles and teaching hospitals are often pictured as aloof, having much higher education, are more skilled, have much more power within the profession, and have no more than a passing concern for private practice doctor's problems, because they have their own battles to fight.

3. The general attitude of "You need me, I don't need you."

4. The academic group has been given the position of leadership in the medical profession for many deserved and earned reasons. Living and practicing daily in such an environment has great educational advantages over private medical practice.

5. There are private practice physicians who are doing the same procedures, have the same talents and skills as those in academic medicine but don't get the notoriety, accolades, prestige, and earnings that the academic group receives. However, some private practicing doctors have found ways to compensate financially for this situation.

Doctors have evolved into becoming paid participants with pharmaceutical and medical instrument companies in their promotions of their products, which presently are being scrutinized and investigated by government agencies. Are there illegal kickback issues here?

For example, the "self-referral" legal loophole is a good example of how doctors have taken to joining other doctors to earn money on the side. By law what they are doing is legal (WSJ, Oct. 23, 2014), but to the government, it's violating the intent of the (Rep. Democrat, California) Pete Stark law passed two decades ago.

Why would doctors go so far as to earn income under risky circumstances by using a legal loophole in the law? According to the WSJ article urologists have been ordering a high-cost diagnostic test for bladder cancer in excessive amounts through a corporate laboratory structure. Doctors who joined the company, 21st Century Oncology, ordered the test through the corporate group lab, which earned the money for the corporation and investors got income back.

This is a good example of what doctors are willing to do to earn extra money while practicing in a fee restrictive environment that's forcing physicians into "professional poverty," as I call it. If doctors never founded a personal outside business for income, as most all doctors never consider doing, and if they know that there is no chance for earning enough money to stay in practice otherwise, why wouldn't they take risks for income gain using every opportunity available to do so.

In my estimation, these risky income producing ventures are snapped-up because they have no alternative in their mind. That alternative is to be fully educated in business principles and strategies, but no one told them about it. No one was compassionate enough to push the business knowledge topic to them earlier in their careers. Accepting risk is what every practicing doctor fully accepts, so risky money-producing efforts are no challenge.

The usual and hard to dismiss comeback from academic physician's response to the under-paid private medical doctors is "You could have done the same thing, but you chose a different life in private medical practice in your medical career." Envy and comparisons do exist.

Probably the best common example of this "elevated" position can be found in the magazines published by any medical school or university system. The physicians featured throughout the magazines are always the doctors who are members of, or connected to, the medical education system in one way or another.

The question to be asked is, "Have you ever personally known of a physician outside this academic medical system (say that he or she is an alumnus of their medical school and is in private practice somewhere doing great things for his or her community), featured in your medical school publications." I haven't. Why not?

One might even incorrectly get the idea that any physician who graduates from medical school and moves to private medical practice has very few, if any, personal medical career accomplishments to offer. At least medical accomplishments that are never important enough to be even mentioned in their own medical school publication sometime during their careers.

I know what you're thinking right now about what I just said. "I'm the most victimized doctor who never received the recognition I deserved from my medical school. Or there exists in me an overwhelming envy of those who are selected for such honors and therefore have a personal complete lack of self-esteem regarding my life in medicine."

Sometimes I do think about these issues, but really don't dwell on them. I think of it as wondering how my career would have turned out if I had chosen some other path to follow. That's because in my career I have received more accolades than most doctors in private practice that I know, which are more than enough to quench my thirst for more attention to my importance.

In my view of the whole medical system, I see areas that must be disturbing to a lot more doctors than me, like the topic of this treatise.

I apologize to those who may be offended, but I prefer to think it is just a matter of different opinions.

My experience has been that those who are offended are commonly those who feel the medical education system is perfect and doesn't need to be changed. They also are those who see problems that could be fixed and say and do nothing about it. There must be literally thousands of those.

6. Employed physicians are often thought of, wrongly, as those doctors at the bottom of the totem pole who didn't have the caliber for private practice or for the academic world.

   These are physicians who are forced to respond to their personal circumstances and are victims of their circumstances unlike physicians in the other two groups. Most become indoctrinated into the "employment-cult" and lose their inspiration to do anything better.

   They learn to believe that their way of practicing as an employee can readily be rationalized as what they were meant to do all along and didn't realize it earlier. So, they are never able to release themselves from the bondage, as restrictive as it is.

Summary-Comments

By putting all of these pieces of information together, one can understand to a reasonable degree why the medical profession has never been able to stand effectively against the various imposing forces.

This also supports the thought that there are ways and means for the medical profession to upgrade itself to a power position that all the resources of the AMA have not yet been able to make happen.

That upgrade, as this physician sees it, is to start at the ground level, even as far back as the premed red-zone. The ability of every doctor should be improved individually to achieve a much higher level of satisfaction, income, and family lifestyle rather than to waste time trying to combat the overwhelming forces we can never overcome.

These forces are:

1. Government control of healthcare

2. Bureaucracy and traditions of the medical profession hierarchy

3. The legal powers and influence dominated by the legal profession within our political system (ex. stalemated medical malpractice reform regarding caps on jury verdicts).

My personal experience as a result of communications with my own classmates about the radical changes happening in the medical profession over at least the last seven decades was a rude awakening for me.

My rather naïve view about the probable future persistence of the camaraderie among and with my classmates while in medical school was wishful thinking.

After having a discussion with my closest friend and classmate in the profession about the major issues all doctors in the private practice of medicine today are facing, it became quite clear to me that my friend was completely oblivious to what was actually happening outside of his forty-some years of academic oriented medical practice.

I also discovered that his views are widely held throughout the medical academic community in which he practiced.

Here were two experienced medical doctors with focused attention on two completely different views about the best way medicine should be headed and how healthcare should be delivered.

Physicians who practice within the academic environment for their whole medical career are:

1. Are mentally comfortable about accepting almost any form of socialized medicine. That's because they are conditioned to living on a stable salary and practicing within an environment that requires almost no business challenges to their practices, someone else takes care of all that.

2. Believe that they are in control of their careers, but have no real idea about how much they are being used as a sacrificial lamb for the benefit of those above them who set the rules they practice under. Just as our government intends to do with the medical profession and has already made great headway in the process.

3. Are practicing within a tight-knit organization community that protects them ferociously; it's something private practice doctors wish they had.

This is just a scenario pointing out the great distance that exists between these two factions of medical practice. This split enhances the need for private practice physicians to be business educated.

Private practice physicians don't have the luxury of "big brother" protecting them, with the business of their medical practice automatically being done for them, and are left out in the open to defend themselves.

This takes us back to the *obligation of medical schools to provide a business education of all medical students*. No matter where a new doctor starts practice after graduation, there is no certainty about their remaining in the same medical practice environment, type of practice, or place of practice for the rest of their medical career. Business knowledge always provides for much more reliable decision-making when changes have to be made.

The anticipated changes that predictably will be forthcoming in our healthcare system can be ameliorated significantly if action is taken today.

Explosion of medical knowledge—how to manage it?

The rapid increase in medical knowledge now being taught to medical students has reached a level where medical education will have to be radically altered in structure, presentation, and methodology. The AMA recently made their plea for those improvements.

Everyone involved in the medical education system has no doubt already discussed the issue of limits on how much a medical student can learn in four years of medical school.

It begs the question of how well massive amounts of medical information can be taught with effectiveness, remembered and used appropriately. There must be a limit on the amount of medical information, the time it takes to teach that information, and the selection of information and education topics and courses necessary to produce a competent physician.

There are several ways to manage this task that directly affect the implementation of an academic business education:

1. Organize the medical curriculum in a way *that focuses on the medical specialty* that the student has an interest in pursuing right from the start of medical school. To make such a foundational change in the medical education system will need to be made sometime in the future. It's time to start now. Following are my thoughts about this:

   A. Students would have to choose a specialty they prefer near the start of medical school. For most, it would be an outrageous guessing game at that time in their medical education. I believe there are ways to discover what they already have skills for doing and could be directed towards those areas of medicine: surgical or medical orientation.

   What is so interesting about choosing a specialty is that many new doctors while doing an internship still haven't made up their minds about what specialty they are willing to spend the rest of their careers practicing. By this time they have had miles of exposure to all medical fields, and still aren't sure. Is that any different than pulling a specialty decision out of a hat in the first year of medical school? Their decision can always be changed along the way.

To compensate, med-student education could then be narrowed down to the knowledge required for that single medical specialty, leaving room and time for other desired education, like business.

A reasonable amount of the general medical education taught in medical school is of very little value to the practicing physicians who later practice within a single specialty.

We've all seen what happens once a physician starts medical practice. For the remainder of their careers most physicians make alterations of their medical practices many times, dump the areas of practice they dislike and focus their attention and then expand on the elements of medical care they find fulfilling and enjoyable.

Doctors are always narrowing down their practice one way or another. A business education enables them to accomplish those changes easily. Without a business education few doctors in private practice can afford to cut out areas of their practice. These doctors commonly try to obtain the skills and knowledge for performing more new procedures they love to do instead. It enables them to increase income and cut out areas of practice they dislike, afterwards.

If you look at what happens, doctors are taught a huge amount of medical information and given training of all kinds. They spend the rest of their careers forgetting, disregarding, and chipping off the medical information they find useless.

All the medical data that they might need outside their specialty are either available online, through CME courses, or through consultant referrals and peer advice.

There is a credible side to the idea that doctors do not need to learn everything while in medical school. After all, they continue to learn for the duration of their medical careers.

B. A doctor's optimal career success can only be attributed to both medical and business education. How much a doctor earns and can afford to increase his or her skills and knowledge, how much a doctor can afford to learn about improving his or her business management skills and knowledge, and how much medical educators care about providing both these things, are the defining elements necessary for the maximum accomplishments of every physician.

2. The medical school *curriculum can be extended to five years* to have the time to make room for every educational process.

A. Such a move would increase the cost of education and students' educational debts.

B. Perhaps the later medical specialty education and training can be shortened to compensate for the specialty learning process acquired during medical school when a student is placed into an educational track towards that specialty.

Then, the total time of medical school of five years, plus one year less of specialty training would equalize the costs and educational time involved... and accomplish all in the same time limits.

3. The great advantage of spreading the business education over the full four years of medical education makes *the implementation process much easier.* Other advantages are as follows:

A. Enables cyclic looping of the business education course including live lectures several times over the four-year education.

B. Various new, revised, or updated segments of the business education can be inserted into the medical education at appropriate times that will correlate with the area in medicine being taught at the time.

For example, the student may be on a six-week rotation through the cardiac surgery department and may be considering where he would train and later practice that specialty.

An essential ingredient of marketing your medical practice business is to start it in an area that allows for growth and expansion of the practice, enough population density, and patients that would be in need of the medical services that you will offer patients.

This would be the right time to be exposed to the business materials and lectures concerning, for example, the choice of a specific geographical area to set up a medical practice that would allow for high probability of business success.

Details that should be considered as follows:

a. The maximum number of patient referrals to your practice that are possible and likely.

b. The area of the practice location that has a wide array of potential patients one prefers to build a practice on.

c. A nearby industry that employs large numbers of people covered by health insurance.

d. The demographics that are compatible with family desires and interests, recreation, and education opportunities.

"Business + medical" educated students always have the upper hand on this and many other critical business issues relating to medical practice success and survival.

The persistent allegation that seems to escape detection

To all medical school deans and medical school academics:

Because of the decades-long history of the medical education scholars' disregard (meaning they knew and did nothing) of the critically important mutual interdependence between both medical education and business education, it lends credence to the allegation that medical education scholars knowingly and intentionally have been and are now responsible for the decades-long financial failure of thousands of private medical practice physicians.

In addition, medical education scholars knowingly are contributing to a great degree to the present disintegration of private medical practice in our nation today. That fact is now playing out, by any reasonable analysis, as a formidable ally to the political progressive agenda of establishing a nationalization of American healthcare.

That issue in turn guarantees that the quality of medical care will decrease and that the full value and maximum professional potential of every medical doctor from now on will be limited to whatever medical care can be delivered in the shortest possible time that meets the requirements that are politically established and dictated by doctor employers.

A message to those who think that they have done enough to streamline the medical education of doctors/students:

Medical education academics, scholars, authorities, decision-makers, and others who honor the integrity of the medical school education system in our nation need to take a step back and make a sincere effort to legitimize in their own minds why the business education of medical students has been neglected for so long, especially when the necessity is so obvious.

Truly understanding that business education is just as important to the lives and professional value of every medical doctor today is a rich and mind-refreshing experience that brings intellectual clarity and wisdom to the topic.

There are a million physicians practicing today in this nation who would gladly celebrate the decision to create and implement a business education for all medical students.

Predictably, you will not find one medical doctor today who has ever practiced medicine in the world of private medical practice that would disagree that an academic business education would have helped them during their medical practice careers.

It's time now to do something about providing an academic business education to all medical students!

Get your scholarly heads together, make a plan to do it, and persist in the effort to make it happen. The objective is not impossible, nor even difficult.

The problem is not that a business education wouldn't help doctors, but that it would disturb the tradition and outdated beliefs of academic minds that lack the skill of present-day entrepreneurial thinking.

You might want to describe this as a revolutionary improvement in training and education of medical doctors/students. It will more than meet the demands of patients, the competition in medical practice, the prime alternative and defense (at present there is none) against restricted fees and controls, and the ultimate cure for the severe frustration and disappointment doctors have about medical practice today.

One final comment I make to all of the scoffing doctors having an unshakable confidence in their employed and academic practice positions today.

There will come a time in medicine when you will be intolerably restricted in what you are allowed to do in medical practice to the point where your ethics will be compromised, your practice functions will be dictated to you, and your position will become vulnerable to termination with one day's notice.

So, I ask you, "What will you do next?"

"We are drowning in information and starving for knowledge."

---Rutherford Rogers

CHAPTER 12

The Recommendations

"Recommendations for the Creation and Implementation of an Academic Business Education Curriculum for Every Medical Student"

For anyone who has a commitment to ensure the best, the most complete and beneficial education of physicians for the purposes of preserving private medical practice, preventing the attrition of doctors, improving the quality of physicians, and enabling doctors to reach their maximum potential, there is only one REASONABLE way to make it happen —by following these recommendations.

ON THE PART of professional medical scholars there are no excuses, distractions, higher priorities, or obligations to not provide an academic business education to all medical students at an age when doctors must have and use business knowledge to attain their maximal productivity and potential in the practice of medicine.

Conscience is sufficient grounds for condemnation of medical academic educators because it establishes a framework of right and wrong. It reflects the law of obligation written in their hearts, which ferments in their minds, but until now has gone no further.

Face it—failure to deliver this high-end business educational necessity for all medical students is a perfect downward spiral to walking through the boneyard of one of the most fundamental bastions of lost educational opportunities ever to be uncovered in modern professional medical education.

What's felt in the heart and known to be true, acts as a moral regulator of one's discernment of what is right or wrong for the benefit of all.

This treatise serves to establish a forthright determination for the business education of medical students starting today. It's an "obligation" mandate to resolve the primary cause of attrition of physicians: lack of adequate income.

Second, it's a supreme enticement for the academic decision-makers to swallow their self-imposed restrictions and their unacceptable bond to the educational "groupthink." And it's a foundational move for the "total education" of physicians today from a ***"good enough"*** objective to one of a ***"maximum potential"*** objective. It requires an academic business education being provided while at the medical student level.

"For things to change, you need to change.
For things to get better, you need to get better."
-Jim Rohn

When you ask yourself what the perfect time is to present an academic business education to potential doctors, there is no better answer than to provide it to all medical students *at the peak time of educational involvement and mental concentration in medical education.*

Educators should not be a stumbling block in the path of all physicians desiring maximum success and accomplishments in their professional careers. Today, they certainly appear to be.

"If you have a *poor* financial education,
you will always work for the rich."
-Robert Kiyosaki

Recommendations for implementation

1. **Create and implement an academic business instruction course** to be required and given to all medical students starting today.

It requires determination and entrepreneurial passion to improve our national healthcare and the physicians' place in that environment regardless of cost, opposition, barriers, or traditional medical education inflexibility.

2. **Inspire all medical education scholars to enlighten and amplify their personal responsibility** that they have appropriately pledged to all medical students and their medical careers.

   Inclusion of an academic and structured formal business education implies that medical education scholars recognize the absolute demanding importance of this *business education issue.*

   Beyond that, there is its *importance to peak medical career competence and accomplishments of every physician*, even without mention of the benefit to our nation's healthcare problems.

3. **We are in desperate need of an open, expressed acknowledgement by the medical academic community that appropriate academic business knowledge of physicians is an intricate and necessary element** required for peak medical career competence, potential, and medical career success today, regardless of any form of opposition.

4. **There needs to be recognition that the provision of such a business education of medical students is the responsibility of medical school academics to arrange for and implement into the education curriculum**, and not the responsibility of another outside business education entity or the medical student themselves.

5. **Take advantage of maximum marketing efforts and opportunities using the business education matrix to expand the prestige and positioning of your medical school's value and educational integrity.**

   By expanding this unique business educational opportunity into the medical education process, every school will have and maintain an empowering recruitment advantage over other medical schools.

6. **An academic business education infrastructure should be created** to meet the variable special focus and goals of each individual medical school.

7. **Academic business education materials and lectures should be offered to students in multiple formats** over the four-year medical education process.

   The teaching process should include live lectures and digitally produced information and materials made available to students 24/7.

8. **It would be advisable to ask all medical education teachers, instructors, and professors to attend the business education lectures and use the digital teaching materials for their own benefit.**

   The probability is that over 95 percent of these educators have never received an academic business education anytime in the past themselves. So, how could they teach it?

   Other medical school instructors and supporters of business education for medical students should be invited to participate in the learning process for free, because the (cost-free) marketing effect of doing that would be highly beneficial to the institution.

9. **This business education strategy, by being "in house," is a much less expensive, more effective, and much more controllable (content and presentation factors) than completely outsourcing the task from the beginning to the end.**

   The greatest advantage to medical schools that do this is that the business program is being implemented into an already exciting and effective medical education curriculum process.

10. **The academic business education materials should be created by business experts** who are very familiar with the business issues faced by private medical practice physicians.

11. **The major goal of medical school business education (of medical students) effort should be to save the *private medical practice of medicine* from complete extinction.**

    Business education will enable all physicians to use that knowledge to maintain and improve their financial stability in spite of the increasing restrictions being placed on the practice of medicine today.

12. **Medical schools starting today should develop a business education curriculum for medical students** that do not directly interfere with the normal medical education process.

13. **Medical schools should begin researching the resources, funding options, and expertise** available or necessary to implement such a business education for medical students.

14. **The "business education system" once created can be marketed** and sold as a product to other medical schools who decide not to try to re-invent the wheel.

15. **Medical schools should create a marketing campaign directed to all premed college programs** detailing the necessity of a business education background (as much as possible) while in college. This campaign would serve as a "mental message" to premed students that business knowledge is very important to medical practice.

    It would also have the effect of affording some degree of necessary business requirements for success before reaching medical school.

    That would make it much easier to teach medical students business principles and inspire them to accept the academic business program once they are in medical school (something that is absent now in nearly all premed programs).

16. **Pressure on premed curriculum administrators** to improve their interactions with premed students through much more detailed information about medical practice business problems resulting from lack of a solid business education. What's needed

are real-life doctors exposing their business problems and solutions, or students will assume that it is all hype, B.S., or an unnecessary college overload.

17. **It's mandatory to alter the *traditional* medicine attitudes about not needing a business education by providing inescapable existing proof to the contrary.**

    Understanding that the "old guys" have fixed opinions and beliefs about medical education that served them well in the last century is entirely inappropriate for today's business world. It may be a clue as to why an academic business education of medical students has consistently been ignored (a misplacement of responsibility).

    Worse yet, these academics wrongly assumed that it was the responsibility of the student to acquire business education sometime later or that it was "somebody else's" responsibility.

18. **Effort should be made to encourage members of the medical school teaching staff to validate the necessity and importance of a business education in the public eye** whenever the opportunity presents itself.

    Absence of any stimulus for a business education of medical students from the teaching staff contributes to the assumption by students that "it isn't needed."

19. **A system for close follow-up, surveys, and statistical analysis of the resultant business education of medical students must be established** over the long term of their private medical practices.

    Any program has to have a means for measuring the parameters of results to be accepted as proof of the effectiveness of the business education. Those results must be compared with private medical practices where the medical students never received a formal business education to demonstrate the difference and the realistic value of a formal business education of physicians.

20. **A fifth year of medical school eventually should be worked into the medical education process.** In view of the current ability for medical students to avoid an internship year and go directly into a residency program, there is acceptable room to create a fifth year of medical school.

    A few medical schools now have a fifth year available to medical students for more advanced education, so the traditional four-year curriculum has already been superseded. This would also provide a time for a more concentrated business education course that might be more effective for learning and remembering the essentials for business success.

21. **A separate investigation into the possibility for the credentialing this formal business education as an authentic MBA program** for all students who complete the required business course. Combined degrees have been offered in medical schools at least since 1958 (MD + PhD).

You likely can add several more to this list of recommendations. These are the most important ones that seem to be within the reach of medical schools grasp and implementation should they choose to update their medical educational curriculums.

We all are aware that new changes in most everything seem easy to begin with, but quickly become hard to accomplish.

"We are all faced with great opportunities brilliantly disguised as impossible situations."
-Charles Swindoll

"If a businessman invested one hour every day doing nothing but thinking, brainstorming, creating new and better ways to be of greater and more valued service to his customers, money problems would melt away."
-Earl Nightingale

CHAPTER 13

The Follow-up

"Physicians: How to Make Today's Forced Revolution in Healthcare and Your "Reactive Response" to Those Forced Changes in the Medical Profession, Work to Your Advantage—Good Business Know-how is Key"

Your choice as to how you adapt to evolving healthcare changes as well as the remaining options left to practicing physicians must be "offensive" in nature (use of business knowledge), aggressive in substance, and exceptionally well planned. You just need to know what options offer the most profitable and tolerable advantages to your medical career.

WITHOUT A DOUBT and whether you believe it or not, your options that are open to your being able to afford to continue in private medical practice demands that you be very well educated in business knowledge and marketing strategies.

The impact of political control of healthcare, economic instability worsening, and the ever-increasing commoditizing of medical practice professionals is so overwhelming that it won't decrease in its effects on every physician predictably for decades to come.

It means not only will it be necessary to adapt to these unfortunate events, but physicians in every mode of medical practice must be far more diligent in their careers than ever in history.

Diligence in your selection of advantageous medical practice options will enable you to reach your most important goals, not all of them.

First, you learn those options, and second, you factor in every desire and objective you have for your medical career. Last, you match them up and make your decisions.

The process will require you to make decisions when you are not ready before you are completely satisfied with your choices and even if the options you discover are the best for you seem wrong at the time.

But, don't worry. The choices you make are a product of both subconscious and conscious experiences, memories, and factors working in your favor. Your mind is smarter than you think. It's called intuition, fueled by the entrepreneurial spirit that doctors are gifted with.

Trends in the medical profession that will influence physician's career decisions far more than anything else…

The most significant trend we see today in the medical profession is the financial failure of private medical practice resulting from lack of ability of doctors to keep their offices open. The classic example of this phenomenon is widely demonstrated by hospitals that are sucking up private medical practices by the thousands across this nation.

Physicians with financial medical practice problems believe that selling their practices to local hospitals and becoming an employee of the hospitals is ultimately better and more sensible than to restart a medical practice in a new location.

The second most obvious trend is the flow of over 50 percent of all graduating medical students out into employed positions, not because they like the idea, but because of the huge educational debt they owe and must start paying back shortly after their training is completed.

Full payback of these loans is nearly impossible, at least for the first five or more years after starting a private medical practice. And after that, the practice must produce enough discretionary income to make the loan payments consistently.

Coupling these two trends should tell you that private medical practice is probably doomed, or at least restricted to physicians with other sources of income or money. Concierge-cash only modes of private medical practice may shortly well become the only leftover element of private medical practice… if we think realistically.

Expanding on that reality a bit, even concierge physicians will be doomed to financial failure of their private practices for a few profound practice-killing reasons...

1. **No business education.**

   Private practices over the last thirty years have been failing for financial reasons and today in increasing numbers. It's all because private practices are run by physicians who were never taught the principles of business required to be successful.

   How could anyone reasonably expect doctors to be highly efficient and productive in medical practice using trial-and-error tactics? Over 95 percent of doctors today, and in the past, suffer from this business education handicap. It has been depriving doctors of the just fruits of their labors for generations.

2. **Formal business education has never been taught or offered to medical students.**

   Every medical school (about 170 of them in the USA) know the necessity of a business education for all doctors, but continue to refuse to take responsibility for providing it to students.

   Leaving that responsibility to the medical students and later physicians to obtain it themselves, has proven to be an embarrassing myth and overly-optimistic prediction.

3. **Medical schools have no intention to provide students with an academic business education (an unacceptable factor).**

   Why have they taken such a stand against something that comprises at least half of the absolute essential ingredients necessary for the optimal success of every private medical practice today?

   Also, ask yourself why they would intentionally reject such an important part of the physician's education process that today is primarily responsible for the financial failure of hundreds, maybe thousands, of private medical practices annually in our country?

   In case you think this is an exaggeration on my part, I suggest you should consider the facts about the reasons that hospitals are rapidly buying up so many medical practices today.

> You must recognize that any physician today sells his or her private medical practice to a hospital for one reason only: The medical practice is not able to financially survive for lack of adequate income or perhaps enough income to compensate the physician appropriate to their status and expectations.

Now that I've stirred up the hornet's nest that puts a twist in the pants of every medical educator reading this, combined with exposing the truth about a major gap in the medical education process, it will either initiate positive action towards providing students with a business education that they must have or they will totally disregard any approach to resolve the issue (as they always have).

Regardless of the response I receive, both myself along with huge numbers of world renowned business educators, consultants, and experts who also agree about the importance of a business education for all medical professionals, will be satisfied.

We have the satisfaction of making an attempt to shake-up the medical education hierarchy about their moral and ethical responsibilities towards all medical students and for providing them with a formal business education.

A diligent look at the medical education system regarding medical schools and medical student education problems…

The unsettling nature of the present ACA and its continued existence, which allows governmental control of our nation's healthcare, doesn't allow any form of stability to be established in the medical profession. Everything, it seems, is either being changed on a weekly basis depending on the whims of a rogue president outside the rule of law and overriding the public majority opinion.

In spite of the medical profession chaos growing out of this environment, the opportunity and necessity to restructure the direction of medical education and medical school curriculums is surfacing faster than expected. The opportunity to shake off old dogmas about medical education is here and now. Predictably, there will likely not be another such opportunity to do this in the future.

When and if complete government control of the healthcare becomes a rigid reality as expected, the secondary effects of that will without a doubt certainly lead to full control of the medical profession.

It won't be simply what they control now, like the regulation of medical doctor licensure, appointed medical boards that enforce government regulations of medical practice, state laws governing the practice of medicine, and government mandates that essentially now control our national hospital system by using economic sanctions.

Up until now, government controls of the medical education system have been primarily economic in nature. Whenever the government hands out taxpayer's money to hospitals, medical schools, and higher education facilities, strings are attached. These entities slowly become dependent on those monies and lock themselves up with the alpha dogs who essentially own them.

I clearly see a time in the near future when all medical schools will be required to follow the same medical school educational curriculum, hospital residency programs, and medical practice regulations. It is nothing more than how labor unions control the workforces in our nation. If you don't join or comply with our rules, you're out.

For non-employed physicians, for example, it means medical licensure anywhere in the USA can be abolished anytime for any reason. Everything becomes a matter of a subjective decision by some bureaucrat who is completely ignorant of how the practice of medicine works most efficiently. Employed physicians already practice under those conditions.

Nothing could have been more predictable than what we see happening today in healthcare and the practice of medicine. But stop licking your wounds because the war isn't over yet.

All it needed was a trigger to make it a permanent circumstance. The trigger was "armed" by entitlements, "cocked" by the political progressive agenda, and "pulled" by the elective support of ignorant and easily misled voters who are addicted to the "freebies" system.

A futuristic view of the future of the medical profession…

All governments organize the various components of their societies into departments for efficiency, subordination, and direct control. We know it in our country by the name of Department of Health and

Human Services (DHHS). One director is appointed to the leadership position and is responsible for everything good and bad that happens within that department and out in the population under the control and approval of the director.

Under this system of government control lays unlimited opportunity to extend its power, which all governments do. It's not difficult to see a time when medical schools will be forced to restrict their teaching activities and curriculums to one or another medical specialty area of education and training.

If a prospective medical student wants to specialize in chest surgery, that student will be sent to a medical associated college that prepares premed students for surgery careers. Upon graduation from college, the student will go directly to the medical school that focuses primarily on surgical education and training or to a medical school that concentrates on chest surgery education alone.

Medical schools would likely be given a choice about what medical specialty they would prefer to focus their attention on or maybe what they already are noted for doing the most and best training of.

Students would essentially be placed out of high school on a single medical career track already established and move up the line of schools they will be required to attend, even the residency program they will already be committed to; they will have no choice of schools or of specialty once they are attached to their career track program.

This kind of education structure would eliminate premed competition between colleges and universities, avoid the necessity of teaching medical students an overwhelming amount of medical information, and likely would produce many more competent and trained physicians than we have now.

There would be hundreds of other problems to resolve connected to this system which can't be fully discussed here.

How does a business education fit into all this?

If we were to assume that the medical education system remained as it is now, we would expect to see graduating medical students increasingly selecting employed positions until it reaches a time when approximately 95 percent of all medical students will do the same.

That would leave about 5 percent (or less) of medical students who either had no educational debts to pay off or had other financial resources to start a private medical practice. There are always a few diehards left who will choose private practice.

"Private" medical practice can be categorized in several forms.

1. Private solo usual medical practice
2. Private group usual medical practice
3. Private solo and group cash-only practice

The 5 percent group of private medical practioners will all be faced with financial problems that will test their very existence, even more so than today. Even today, private physicians are having major financial problems that are already for them irresolvable.

The only opportunity for all these doctors to survive in solo or group private practices is to start medical practice armed with an academic business education. The only practical and realistic time for that business education to be implemented is while they are still in medical school, as has been well documented over the past several decades by less than 1 percent of physicians ever doing it on their own.

On the other hand, it would seem that employed physicians would have very little reason to obtain a full business education. In most cases the employer-owners manage the business elements of the medical practice for them and take their cut of the income created by the physicians.

For the majority of the new generation physicians, who are core focused on their profession as a means of financial gain high enough to meet their immediate needs, pay off their educational debts, and leave enough time off for family and personal ventures.

As an employed physician, they know that they can embrace all those advantages to the fullest.

"Employed" medical practice is divided as follows:

1. Medical practice as a solo employed physician
2. Medical practice as a group of employed medical providers
3. Private (solo and group) contracted medical practice

However, there are a few factors that tend to directly interfere with those desirable advantages and that may well throw them back into the difficult financial bin with the private practice doctors.

About 10-15 percent of employed physicians eventually default in that role, for one of many reasons…

1. **Conflicts with the system…**

   Because of my fourteen years of my medical practice in three different medical systems of practice, I can tell you that I have heard most of the most common reasons that those physicians had for leaving the system, including my own.

   I found that the most common reason they left was because of some type of practice restrictions. You must understand that each system of medical practice is established primarily for profit reasons… businesses have to make a profit to pay overhead, employees, and business essentials, as well as to continue growing.

   Growth is necessary to survive the business competition, inflation of the economy, and economic gain that perpetuates the cycle.

   Physicians as employees become pons for manipulation by the system. It means that the employers set the medical performance rules for what you are expected to accomplish. The rules are established to effectively increase a doctor's income productivity, not his or her salary or benefits.

   Medical functions, processes, and procedures that doctors are knowledgeable about and trained to do competently, doctors may not be allowed to do.

   If medical practice issues are believed by the business/employer to be *unessential to the welfare of the patient* or don't provide enough income for the time spent with it, and the doctor's time is much more profitable doing something else in place of it, then you will be forbidden to do it.

   That's why presently psychiatric care, infertility procedures, medical consulting with patients, are commonly forbidden. On some occasions those things will be relegated to mid-level providers with less knowledge and experience. It also is a cheaper means of temporarily complying with the overall health mandates by looking like they are providing more inclusive health services.

You can easily understand what it does to a doctor that comes out of medical training supercharged to make a difference in the world using everything they have learned to do competently, then being told they can't do all that important stuff with your new ideas and talents.

Just out of my residency and financially broke, I began my career at Kaiser Permanente. I couldn't wait to show everyone around me what I was capable of doing in medical practice. I thought that being able to speak out at the department meetings about what I had recently learned about treating patients and their problems would be refreshing and educational to the other members. Boy, was I wrong.

Not only was I "put down" by the senior members of the department for being a bragger and know-it-all for offering comments at meetings, but they required that I be taken aside by a friendly senior department member and informed about how not to irritate the others in the department who didn't want a young smart-ass lecturing to them. So, I complied. You know, "When in Rome..."

Just being able to do all the everyday routine money producing medical procedures and work is all they want from you. Think you might become a robot on the medical provider assembly line? Some can live with that; some can't.

However, there are some advantages to that scenario. You don't have to think hard. You don't have to increase your medical or technical expertise at all, even for years. Keeping up in your specialty advancements is easier because you likely will not be allowed to do those procedures or see those needful patients anyway. They are "referred out" to outside experts.

Besides, they're on a rigid budget from above and may not be able to buy the equipment or technology for a few years. If you are the only doctor to use the equipment and procedure... then, forget it.

As you might imagine, clamping down on a person's mind-power, intentions, desires, passions and expectations quickly leads to loss of passion to practice, loss of desire to do more than is expected of you, and loss of self-esteem because you are not in control of your career… the employer is.

For physicians who continue maintain those values, it becomes a priority to move to a practice mode where those attributes can be manifested.

2. **Restrictions on their practice functions and beliefs…**

This reason for seeking a new and different practice mode where you are in total control of your life and career is no doubt the most powerful cause to leave an employed position as a physician—at least it was for me.

The natural instinct of every graduating physician is to follow their intense desire to use and expand on almost every aspect of their medical knowledge, training, and talents as soon as possible. At that time, the motivation to earn money takes second place in their thoughts.

I won't tell you about my experience with my hospital job except to mention my use of my OB ultrasound machine. I took my own ultrasound machine (six years using it) with me to my new hospital job at their Women's Clinic in MI when I discovered that all the staff OB-Gyn doctor's (ten) on the medical staff had never been trained to use an ultrasound device in their OBG practices. I thought I could get them interested in getting one.

After two months of using my ultrasound on my own patients in the clinic, I was *ordered* not to use my ultrasound at all on any patients, even to demonstrate its use. The reason: Radiology department would lose money by my doing my own ultrasounds. I never billed for the procedure. I used it to improve my diagnostic accuracy and avoid missing something that I couldn't feel on pelvic examination.

Several other disturbing events followed after that at the hospital. It began when I moved from my California practice, where OBG ultrasound use was widespread and operative laparoscopy was many years old, to a Midwest state and hospital that surgically was ten years behind current medical practice procedures.

The hospital had never developed a surgical privileges list for operative laparoscopy, so I had them copy the one I brought from California.

After their investigation, I was gratefully given those advanced medical and surgical privileges. The operating room supervisor informed me that they already had all the latest operative laparoscopic equipment. What she meant was that they had all the equipment for laparoscopic tubal ligations, nothing above that.

After attempting an operative laparoscopic procedure that I had done in California many times, the lack of appropriate instruments forced me to manage the case in an open procedure. This doubled my surgical time slot and knocked a couple other surgeons off the OR schedule because of the time I used up and later apologized for. I agreed not to do any advanced laparoscopic procedures for the rest of my contract time there, primarily for my own benefit.

It was a matter of scrubbing on cases without proper instrumentation, without trained assistants and nurses for those procedures, and to avoid the consequent risks associated with those deficiencies.

The shame of it was that they had a highly qualified and experienced surgeon on staff at their doorstep that could have helped them to upgrade the competence of the surgical staff, at least those who wanted to upgrade their skills.

It goes without saying that the publicity of such skills would have drawn more patients, more qualified medical staff, and maximized the hospital profits in the process. Leadership without a futuristic view of healthcare trends and improvement strategies maintains stagnation.

Any of the ten OB-Gyn doctors with a business education could have taken this one surgical skill and dominated the local market for those kind of patients for years to come, but they never did while I was there, and never asked me to help them or teach them anything.

I left when they did not renew my contract. It took me a long time to understand that one of the reasons for their action was that I did not meet the patient visit quotas that other clinic doctors (OBG) there had established as the norm; either see and treat at least sixty patients a day in the clinic, or be replaced. I wasn't earning the hospital enough money. Does that ring a bell about what I told you above about an employee's obligation to be productive enough?

I forgot to mention that the previous Kaiser HMO told me I was not allowed to do infertility work on patients. No health insurance paid for it because it was voluntary and not an essential healthcare issue.

3. **Changes in their career priorities…**

The natural freedom physicians feel and that inspires their passion to squeeze every drop of knowledge and creativity out of their minds and into what they know and do in medical care, is a very difficult emotion to harness. Only when they are forced to personally suppress that intense desire can any physician survive within an employed position.

Regardless of a physician's seeming adaptation to the doctor's life in captivity, each one is always looking for a means to reach a higher level of medical practice freedom, consciously or unconsciously.

At least one in ten medical doctors reach a tolerance level as an employee that is incompatible with their dreams and expectations, and they have to leave their employee-ship servitude.

What provides financial fulfillment can rarely override the fulfillment of medical practice freedom. If financial rewards do win them over, it means either that there are significant external factors driving them such as family needs, or there are personal dependency aspects of their personality that override their decisions and actions.

In these cases, their emotions are fulfilled and are more important to them than their careers. And there is nothing wrong with that.

I discovered from my experiences of employment that there usually is a circumstance in the life of the doctor that triggers the desire to leave their employed position. It's commonly an opportunity that presents itself from outside their employed environment. Either a doctor friend or an old connection with an outside prior medical career experience and person provides the opportunity.

Commonly, the doctor's choice made at the beginning to accept an employed job was because it was a last choice available at the time, or perhaps it was intended to be only a temporary job, which is "addictive."

Anyone who chooses an employed position should be aware that there is about a 10-14 percent chance that they will leave that job in the future for one reason or another. It's smart to have a backup plan for several good reasons you can imagine.

Should you get fired from your job, it usually is quite unexpected and leaves you without a backup plan. When my hospital contract was not renewed, it was totally unexpected.

In my mind, I believed that I had done a medical job worthy of notice and had complied with the hospital demands beyond what most physicians would not have tolerated. The two different physicians that the hospital had hired in sequence for the same position prior to me lasted only a matter of months and quit.

My naive mistake was thinking that doing excellent medical practice was key to my importance as an employee rather than meeting the quota of patient contacts per day that the hospital received income from. If I had had business knowledge, I would have seen it coming long before it happened and prepared.

Today there is no problem for entities to replace you anytime. The waiting list for your job is huge. Keeping all of your outside contacts open along the way is a very important issue for you to protect yourself.

4. **Personal and family life alterations.**

A strong offer from a peer friend to come and practice with him is undoubtedly the number one trigger to leave. It was for me. I knew that I was not happy as an employed physician at Kaiser from the start, but at the time I had run out of choices and was out of money with a wife and two small children we had adopted.

I had befriended a local doctor at a medical society meeting who was busy in practice, overloaded with patients. He agreed to send me loads of patients that he would never be able to handle... and later did exactly what he said he would do.

A couple of months after that, I decided to quit Kaiser because they restricted my infertility work. For example, when you are seeing an infertility patient and tell them to make an appointment to check them during their ovulation time mid-menstrual-cycle a few days later, trouble began. My patient schedule was 100 percent scheduled with medical patients for three months ahead at all times-no openings. Remember, the employer controls all patient-scheduling.

Squeezing that patient into my regular schedule required seeing two patients in that fifteen to twenty minute timeslot or after the usual clinic hours. Both options were forbidden and were reason for dismissal if it continued. It sealed my decision to leave.

Divorce is another problem. Alimony can destroy doctors. At least it causes them to move as far away from their X-marital-partner as possible. One doctor friend chose to work in an Indian reservation clinic two thousand miles away from his X. He earned enough money to live frugally and had none left to meet his alimony obligations (several thousand dollars per month). Many of you understand and have faced the same problems.

Personal health problems can be another determining factor for leaving employed positions. The HMO system is not about to keep a doctor on staff who can't carry his full load of patients. You will be let go regardless of how good a doctor you are. However, if you had had a formal business education, you would be primed to stay on in an administrative position.

A complete change of mind about what you want to do with your medical career is the third most frequent reason for quitting an employed job as a physician.

If you love to teach, love to do research, or enjoy academic life as a physician, finding a position compatible with those interests as an employee are few and far between. If you find one, then you usually need to move your family, kids change schools (which most hate to do), and the whole process is often more of a dilemma than staying in a job and living with the consequences.

5. **Realization that your career goals will not be met.**

   Being confined to an employed position nearly always requires a complete change in your career planning because you are no longer in charge of your medical career—they are.

   It's enough of a reason to quit your employed position any time because medical career goals for most doctors often can't be met while in an employed job. It's just the way it is.

   I discovered that those who stay employed for long periods of time often are incompetent, lazy, lack passion, have never had career goals, love their free time more than their commitment to medical practice and career, and/or are doctors qualified only for what advantages employment offers.

   One OBG doctor I worked with came from a very wealthy family and couldn't do an endometrial biopsy procedure, probably one of the safest uncomplicated surgical office procedures in gyn care today. He refused to do any OB or any major surgical procedures, but was very good at seeing clinic patients rapidly.

   He existed in his job because the other OBG doctors continued to be willing to always help him out with his patients, and he required lots of help.

The future value of a formal business education of medical students in a nationalized healthcare system...

If one takes the position that all physicians will eventually become government employees under the evolving ACA, the necessity of having large numbers of physicians being trained in business as well as in medicine is even more important than ever.

With the predictable and increased use of mid-level medical care providers, physicians will take on more administrative and supervisory roles. Therefore, physicians who have a formal business education background will have a distinct advantage over those who don't.

Another advantage for physicians with a formal business education will be the fact that these physicians will provide more credibility concerning their feedback business advice to administrators who attempt to make efficiency and productivity improvements in the healthcare system. The value of these physicians for the improvement of the business side of the healthcare system will be a valuable asset.

Still another advantage for these physicians is their superior position for any other business job position within the healthcare system and outside the healthcare system. It's reasonable to assume that business-trained physicians add a dimension of value to any business well above other physicians lacking it.

Who wouldn't select a business-educated physician over a physician without that kind of background?

Such a business-educated physician would qualify for a higher salary and benefits as well. It would also be a definite advantage for physicians in the academic world, teaching positions, and medical research work.

There is little doubt that everyone would benefit substantially from a business education because almost every source of income involves some sort of business entity that employees must deal with. Employees with a business background understand why most things in business are done and the reasons for doing them, thus promoting fewer conflicts and disruptions in the workforce.

This admonition about the imperative for a formal business education of all postgraduate professionals can be appropriately applied to dental education as well as legal education students, who also lack any significant business education during their training.

The great business minds, business experts, business educators, and business knowledge experts say…

"I think all persons should be in business for themselves… at the very least working after hours from their day job."

-Dan S. Kennedy, forty years as a serial entrepreneur and teacher of entrepreneurs

"Today's medical schools typically provide minimal instruction about the business of medicine and the way healthcare systems work, but future physicians must be well versed in these topics so they can thrive in rapidly changing settings."

- Ardis D. Hoven, MD, President,
American Medical Association
(*WSJ* Letters to Editor, October 2, 2013)

**"If you can't handle the money,
you can't handle your destiny."**

Reverend Robert Morris, Gateway Church

CHAPTER 14

The Treating Doctor

"The Real Story: How My Business Ignorance Propelled Me into a Second Purpose for My Life and a New Career Destined to Significantly Improve Medical School Education and the Medical Careers for All Physicians"

Sometimes we discover the most important purpose for our lives while we are searching for answers to something completely different.

I HAVE ANOTHER *suggestion and recommendation* for you to benefit from, which often is found to be more inspiring than pages of authoritative text that tries to persuade physicians to do something that they have very little reason to believe or trust.

This story is about my medical practice experiences that resulted in losing my private medical practice. Although there are other less important contributing factors that helped undermine my medical practice financial stability, the most critical one by far was my complete business incompetency about running my medical practice business.

It's not that I didn't try everything that I thought or knew at the time might help to reverse my financial failure-in-progress. It was the fact that I had never learned anything about doing business or running a business.

Yet there I was implanted in a solo medical practice business (after about fifteen years in solo medical practice at the time) of my own choice.

I had no real business understanding that to have a sound business knowledge would have made an astounding difference in the outcome for me and my family. It likely would have never resulted in my writing this book.

The pain: transition to private medical practice.

Beginning private medical practice is always a very stimulating and exciting time for any physician. I had just spent two and a half years at Kaiser Permanente. Being the only one of the twelve OBG physicians there who had any interest in infertility problems, the others pushed all their patients with infertility issues on to me.

It soon became evident there was a clear reason that the other doctors seemed so helpful.

What I didn't know at the time was that the "Kaiser system" was structured to avoid non-profitable medical treatments that used up a considerable amount of doctor-time that could have otherwise been much more profitable for the "system."

I attempted to treat these infertility patients in a very effective manner, frequently squeezing my infertility patients at ovulation time and late cycle in between my other scheduled patients. It resulted in the need to keep my nurse overtime in order to see all my scheduled patients led the Chief of Service to inform me that I was not permitted to foul up the standard working hours like I had been abusing. I was told that money was not allocated to pay nurses for overtime work and I was wasting their money.

The options given me were to comply or leave. I left because I understood that my personal desire to treat infertility patients and to give each of them my unrestricted time and care was far more fulfilling to me than short-changing them of proper care by implementing "Kaiser Care" instead.

After starting my private solo practice locally (about a mile away in the same city) soon after I left with the advice and assistance of a local busy OBG doctor, I found myself mired with a thousand jobs to be done all at the same time. With no income coming in those first few months I continued to work at the Kaiser Clinic to pay our personal and practice bills.

At this time I had absolutely no knowledge about how to manage a private medical practice, but figured I could handle it with some help from other doctors and their office personnel. Back in 1970, no books on the matter were available. But today, I found very few books to read and follow on this topic. The available books on starting medical practice and how to manage a medical practice today spend a lot of content explaining "what" to do and "when." But all that I have read, unfortunately, lack the details of "how" to accomplish the advice being given.

Fortunately, even in the local medical community of doctors, it was rare to find a private OBG doctor who did much infertility work. Health insurance didn't cover infertility care and treatment. So I received many patient referrals for infertility care that helped build my practice faster than I expected, but also handed me a load of poor paying infertility patients whose workup proceeded based on when they could pay.

Over the next few years I could see that my practice income would never reach the level of income necessary (using the borrowed medical practice management information) for funding my retirement plan or paying for my three kids to go through college.

Consequently, I began looking for ways to make more money in my practice and outside the practice. I then did extra jobs that involved working longer and harder like consulting on malpractice cases, real estate investing, taking extra OB "on-call" nights, selling medications in my office through a vendor, etc.

The extra practice income I used to improve my skills and knowledge in OBG thinking that it would pay off eventually, which it did. My new skills that brought in new patients were ones that were new to our specialty like; ultrasound use, IVF, tubal microsurgery, laparoscopy and advanced pelviscopy, advanced fetal monitoring, hysteroscopy procedures, outpatient breast lumpectomies, among others.

I reached the cutting edge of my specialty at the same time that the "managed care mandate" peaked in popularity in the late 1970s.

My medical practice income never significantly increased during all these years because of two practice-killing events that intervened.

First, every medical malpractice insurance company quit selling insurance in California because of the outrageous millions of dollars jury verdicts and awards, primarily from the "pain and suffering" element of the law, and the fact that doctors could not afford the premiums.

I was forced to go "bare" (no malpractice insurance coverage) for about two years until I joined a physician-created malpractice insurance company (CAP-MPT) that sprung up in California after all of the standard malpractice insurers had stopped selling such coverage in California. CAP-MPT advised and I used "arbitration" contracts for protection. Interestingly, I remember that only one patient in my practice during that time refused to sign the arbitration agreement, contrary to the numbers published regarding this important issue.

Second, my patients left to join the doctors and practices that had joined the HMO, PPO, and IPO managed care groups. Employers had contracted with these groups to cover the healthcare of their employees. In these cases patients were forced into a decision; continue with their private practice doctor and pay for everything out of pocket, or use the services of the managed care contracted entity which covered their care.

To stem that patient tide leaving my practice and against my best judgment, I joined every managed care organization I could find—over two hundred of them. That effort failed to maintain my patient volume. None of my old patients returned to my office that I can remember once they were enrolled in the managed care contracts.

By this time, I could see my practice income decreasing continuously in spite of all my attempts to prevent loss of my patients. My depression and physical body problems were increasing and visible to everyone around me.

The severe depression required years of psychiatric care. Later I was diagnosed with "combat PTSD" by the Veterans Administration doctors resulting from my eighty plus combat missions in Vietnam years earlier (1965). Such an approved diagnosis was not valid and not in the official medical diagnosis books prior to 1970.

I had been fighting my battle with depression on my own fairly well since 1965 up until things were reaching the point of being hopeless. I was divorced in 1985 and that was far from helpful. All my immediate family lived three thousand miles away on the East Coast and was not very helpful under those circumstances.

I ran out of income and watched my medical practice disappear from underneath me. Having undergone bankruptcy, suffered through the consequences of a bad obstetrical malpractice case, and living on credit cards completely while living newly married (1989), I finally found (two years of looking) an employed position at a hospital in Michigan that paid well. There, I managed to use all that extra income to pay off all my leftover practice withholding tax I never paid the last few years that my practice continued, all credit card balances, and legal bills from my medical practice and divorce problems.

The one lifesaving event that kept me going was that I had found and married a fantastic lady who was able to see, understand, and encourage me through all my problems, and still does today—almost thirty years later. It had to have happened because of Divine Providence and arrangement. It wasn't simply luck.

Summary: The end of my medical career.

In my mind at the time, I had miserably failed in my career and personal life, which compounded my self-criticism and depression.

At that time I really had no real idea why or how I had lost my medical practice, why I was unable to rescue it, and where to turn to next. I had no backup plan in place (a big mistake) because I never dreamed that such a thing could happen to me.

All that time it seemed to be just some uncontrollable destructive glitches in my medical career that would be over soon and all would return back to normal… and didn't.

I did see the new OBG doctors moving into town and didn't recognize what that competition would do to my medical practice. I just took it for granted that it would all work out OK. In my mind I had no concern that practice competition in my specialty would ever be able to seriously affect or ever destroy the great medical practice I had built over the years.

All I knew was that I didn't have enough money to keep my office open and pay my bills, and had no idea how I would ever improve on my desperate financial situation. In addition, because I could never fathom how I would ever lose my practice in the first place, I had never thought about what would happen if I did lose it until the last few months. It was the first time in my life that I had failed to create a backup plan for my career path.

I had no business judgment about how to measure my patient load and never thought of keeping a log of new patients coming in and old patients leaving. What a dummy I was!

Naturally, I was forced to change everything in my life. Financially, I had to become an employed physician again (I had served in the Navy with Marines for a total of six years earlier and spent over two years at Kaiser Permanente) until I quit medicine in 1999. Because of the malpractice risk factors mentally hounding me daily in OB and my severe distaste of being a controlled employee for the rest of my career, I could not avoid leaving the profession. My fear of restarting a new private practice and failing again was not in my mind a sustainable alternative.

I was angry at myself for not being able to maintain control of my career and for not having the foresight and intelligence to create solutions to my professional problems. My severe daily headaches, irritable bowel syndrome, insomnia, and stress level didn't help either. My wife agreed with my decision to quit medicine.

Another final lapse of my judgment and regrettable decisions I made at the time was that I cut all ties to medicine by canceling all medical licensures I had. That decision has come back to haunt me over and over again. Had I at least continued to maintain one "active" state medical licensure it would have permitted me some medical practice options I could have taken advantage of, should my thoughts and circumstances change.

I could have (if I had had an active medical license in any state)...

1. Restarted a private medical practice later if I changed my mind.

2. Taught medical students and residents at medical schools.

3. Worked part time or full time at a government medical facility such as Veterans medical facilities, hospitals, clinics, or Indian reservation medical centers or hospitals.

My turnaround finally happened...

After I finally quit medicine it took me over two years of sheer boredom and financial problems (I never was able to fund a retirement plan) to realize that God must have another purpose for me. Rather than live on social security checks for the rest of our lives in relative "professional poverty," I had to find something to do to make some money for my wife Linda and I.

I truly had never considered how I would feel emotionally about suddenly not seeing medical patients and going to work every day in medical practice. I had never intended to retire from medical practice.

Then I discovered that I was a person that needed to be doing something productive every day of my life; it was just the way I was as a person with that kind of work ethic.

Because all I really knew much about was medicine, I thought I'd start looking at possibilities in that familiar area. The process became easier in 2000 when I discovered that the Internet had opened the doors to a world of opportunities. Not only were there opportunities worldwide, but I could create a business online and do everything from home on a computer. It sounded good to me because it seemed everybody was doing it and earning money as well. I took the bait.

I created a website and an online retail business to sell camping supplies (we had done a good amount of camping and my wife enjoyed it more than I did). The RV world was alive and increasing among retirees. At this time I still had no knowledge of how to run any business successfully and as you may understand, I made only two sales from my camping website in a year and a half for about $30 total. It didn't match my definition of a successful business. Yep, it was just another failure to stack on top of the previous ones.

However, it was an eye-opening failure that proved to me that creating a profitable business meant learning to use the Internet with the right business knowledge. And more importantly, to be successful online I learned that I would also have to stop everything I was doing and learn about marketing and the common foundational business principles.

I spent the next year becoming fully computer and Internet literate. I also began reading every book about business and marketing success that I could afford. I also discovered hundreds of free newsletters published online by the world experts on both topics, which I subscribed to over time. Included with newsletters were references to hundreds of business and marketing online courses, webinars, teleseminars, and packaged information they sold themselves.

After a few months of studying these very interesting and informative resources, the whole world of how to make a business successful, and manage it in a profitable fashion using the right business tools, I became persuaded that this learning experience was essential to my business future. It was a no-brainer.

As I attended more business and marketing conferences over several years, read more business and marketing newsletters and books by many of the business experts, and boned up on the latest problems in the medical profession today, the increasing attrition of doctors and the decreasing incomes of doctors across the profession ignited a compelling truth in my mind.

Catch-up information pertinent to my story...

A few catch-up factors: After I quit medical practice, I continued to receive medical practice journals, newsletters, alumni medical school news, and continued to hear and read in the media about all the serious medical profession problems surfacing in our country.

This was the time when I began to realize the connection being made in my mind between the increasing attrition and severe nationwide frustration among the majority of physicians today and my previous personal, yet continuing deep desire to figure out why I had lost my own medical practice.

It became a profound revelation to me that there was some unknown yet direct connection between what happened to those many other doctors and what had happened to my practice. Obviously I wasn't the only recipient of practice failure. It was a beautiful feeling to find my mind open to new possibilities and digging for answers.

One day the answer to why I had lost my medical practice came into full view. My medical practice didn't fail because I was a medically dumb doctor, or because of all the disarming circumstances I had faced while in practice. It happened because of my ignorance about the other half of private medical practice... the business side of medical practice, which had remained disconnected from my mind all those years in medical practice.

I had done what 98 percent of other private practice doctors had done to make their practice grow, but I was missing some elements of practice growth that they had done automatically and without business knowledge. Years later I recognized what they did that kept their practices growing and I didn't. Their success was not related to gaining a complete knowledge of business and marketing and implementing that knowledge.

Their success in practice I believe today was their extensive social interactions with everyone in the medical community and participation in nearly all social interactions when the opportunity presented itself. I had no inclination for social interaction or interest in participation in them.

Little did I understand the practice-building value of that issue at the time. Never did I understand that their social activities drew many more patient referrals, consultations, and provided great trust and likeability in the medical and public communities.

Years later, once I had gained enough knowledge about successful business strategies and the value and use of marketing, *I finally knew why I had lost my medical practice* and what I could have done to save it, if I had known or been taught business principles.

I finally understood that my associate's natural inclination for social interactions enabled them to survive without business education. I'm confident today that they had no idea why they had done so well in their medical practice business without having a business education.

Those of us who are introverted and shy away from the medical community interactions in all probability need a business education to use as our means to medical practice survivability and growth. Once one knows the importance of business principles and success, one can compensate for our other personality and communication weaknesses.

When I go into deep thinking about these factors, I believe that had I had a formal business education during medical school, I would have had the ability and tools to overcome my social weaknesses with ease, and would have outperformed the majority of the physicians I knew not only in practice building, but also in practice income in a permanently sustainable fashion during my medical career and life.

It's highly probable that those doctors who had the social graces as well as a business education would have easily outreached all of us.

The breakthrough completely changed my perspective about medical practice…

It was a rude awakening to then understand that my failed medical practice was caused primarily by my lack of a formal business education.

I recognized that my path had to be a total knowledge of all aspects of business functions and principles, not just a confabulation of intermittent injections of happenstance business ideas and bits of business information such as those used by almost all physicians today who start private practices; all this can be considered my "on-the-job training."

Physicians' practices across the country are *financially failing* primarily because they never had the business knowledge to use to survive their practice demise, let alone prevent it. Every physician today knows that all medical practices don't survive, but have very little insight as to the real reason. I doubt that any of them truthfully know the real causes.

After some investigation, I discovered that no medical school in the USA provides or even offers a formal business education to medical students.

What was even more disturbing to me as I looked back was the complete absence of any premed or medical school mention or advice about *the importance of* an *academic business education and the value of it for maximizing private medical practice success.*

I recognized that the direct connection between medical school education and the increasing financial failure of hundreds of medical practices, as well as increasing attrition of doctors today, is the result of an obvious lack of an academic business education.

My mission began even without my own endorsement. It was like the "Pelosi doctrine—we'll pass the health care law and then find out what's in it later." I felt compelled to get the word out, regardless.

With the expertise that I had developed over many years working in business and marketing methods and strategies, I knew that I was one of the few medical doctors today with *both medical practice and business expertise* that enables me to integrate the two at a much more understandable and practical level than most other non-medical business experts.

My purpose became highly focused when…

It was in 2005 when this hit me. I gave up all my other interests that I had been working on regarding an online business. My decision and conviction was then and is now to explain to all who will listen how to avoid financial failure of their medical practices and how to use business knowledge to earn the income needed.

After my literature search and the discovery that Amazon.com had more than 250,000 books listed in the category of business and marketing, I discovered only two books published on business and marketing *for physicians*. Both were published before the Internet hit the scene and have been revised since.

It's rare to find a physician who isn't hurting financially today.

I created a professional medical website focused on teaching these medical practice business processes, tools, and principles.

www.marketingamedicalpractice.com

Six years ago I began a free email newsletter for medical professional subscribers using my own articles to connect every aspect of medical practice improvement with a business and marketing strategy to use to build their own practices. It continues to be my effort to help other physicians survive in private practice, not just as a means to make money enough to raise above the social security rolls.

I had by that time invested a large amount of inherited money in my business and marketing education and believe that my recuperation of invested costs will happen at a later time as my project continues to unfold into creative new avenues of progress.

As of this writing, I have over sixty-five such business and marketing educational articles of mine published online for physicians (actually ones that are very appropriate for any professional medical care provider) listed and available on the website.

These articles are for the educational use by any physician who makes a courageous decision to increase their practice income and their own professional skills and education.

The unique aspects of my educational approach effectively has *at least three cutting edge benefits that presently far surpasses* those rare other professional individuals who have also taken their time to create reliable, highly regarded, and evidence-driven books and guidelines about how to establish, manage, and maintain their private practices.

First, my research, articles, educational materials, ideas, advice, and recommendations are all composed and extracted from a wide range of world-class business and marketing experts who are the highest regarded consultants and business experts in the world today (whether still living or not).

You need to understand that most authors, who write the books and materials about how to improve medical practices...

1. *Rely on their "own" successful medical practice experiences* and the *help of a few other special experts* within the practice of medicine field to create their content which is usually restricted to a small number of business ideas as opposed to a world of experts that I rely on daily.

   Remember: Physicians who write these books to help other doctors *rarely have had a formal education in business themselves* and so they rely on co-authors (non-physicians) to do the business education part. These non-physician business experts are commonly unable to reach the depth of medical practice functions where the real problems occur and physicians need help with.

2. These authors, understandably, focus their attention on their personal experiential ideas and information about what they consider are the most important topics and advice medical students and young doctors have the greatest need for.

   The problem with that information is that it usually is from people who have great experience behind what they say and believe, but often comes from expert business specialists who have **not** *spent a career dealing primarily with medical doctors* and helping them with their medical practice problems.

3. Other authors spend additional time writing about how to obtain medical licensure, set up an office practice, and buy the right equipment needed. They provide lists of medical regulations that must be followed, and spend much *less time about personally managing the medical practice.*

   Most authors tend to suggest that it is *better to rely on outside experts* in each area of an office practice business setup process, which is a cost most doctors can't afford at a time when they have no job, have large debts to pay, and have great difficulty obtaining loans.

4. You'll also notice that the authors of these books tell readers what needs to be done and very little about how to do it, primarily because it would take an inordinate amount of time to explain it properly in a book format.

   A related issue is that of *medical practice management* and *management of the business of medical practice.* The specifics of both segments of private medical practice are rarely discussed in detail, which I believe to be of great importance. Failure to know how to achieve these two critical management requirements is the *primary cause of financial failure* of private medical practice today and has been for the last six decades at least.

Second, there is a common assumption that what is being taught about business by college and university professors and in business schools is not only top-of-the-line business information, but are also the principles and procedures that are essential for the success of any business.

However, if you speak to a medical student today who entered medical school recently and who already has an MBA degree, you will quickly discover as I did that what they learned in business school was far from being of much help to them regarding medical practice business. Why?

What's missing here?

The connection between the practical and usual business education and the business of medical practice is extremely fragile based on *one very important factor* that rarely reaches the ears of those who teach business at the graduate level.

That factor can be described as an educational necessity, in the case of graduate professionals such as physicians or medical students, of bonding or interlacing the business lessons directly (at the same time) with actual practical medical practice business problems that all doctors in private medical practice face.

The reason that this intermixing is so important is that the medical students and doctors just starting their practices have absolutely no knowledge about what business problems they will later face in actual practice.

It's similar to teaching someone how to construct a personal computer, with the intent that sometime in the future they may need to know how to use it. If they are taught how to use a computer while they are learning to build one, their motivation and effort to learn and remember is significantly magnified.

If a medical student somehow experiences real problems that doctors actually have in medical practice while they are learning medical business principles and strategies focused on medical practice, they will more readily retain that knowledge associated with the business experience in memory.

Otherwise the book and lecture learning will quickly be forgotten, disregarded, or ignored. When one sees the real reasons for learning something, they comply.

These are the reasons that a formal business education must be taught at the same time while medical students are still in medical school. It's also a great part of why doctors never later stop to obtain a business education, even when they know that it would undoubtedly help them.

Third, what I teach and advise goes far beyond the standard everyday business principles that apply to virtually all successful businesses. What does vary is how one applies those principles and strategies to each different business. *How they are applied to one medical practice differs entirely from all other medical practices.*

The applications of business strategies, tactics, and objective intentions are different for every physician in private medical practice. It follows that the creation, structure, and ultimate use of these business tools, in order to accomplish the goals of each individual medical doctor, have to be applied and implemented in a manner that enables each doctor's objectives to be met.

The application of *general* business standards, principles, and rules, on the other hand, are inadequate to accomplish the specific diversified desires of each physician in each medical practice.

The ultimate basic challenge of a formal business education of medical students (or physicians) is to teach the basics of business and marketing before moving to the next higher level of specific business education.

The higher and essential challenge of a physician's business education is to provide guidelines for physicians to use that can be specifically used as a template to accomplish their personal goals for their medical practice and medical career.

So far, in our present medical practice world of physicians, this kind of business education of physicians and medical students doesn't exist, but must exist if medical scholars and educators intend to preserve private medical practice in our elite society.

My intentions…

What I've learned and that I teach comes directly from business experts who completed the gauntlet between "starting-from-scratch" to building highly successful business enterprises, as opposed to business school professors who teach the information and have never done it themselves. The quality and practical usefulness of their teachings are too general in nature to be of more than menial value to physicians (even to other medical professionals such as dentists).

Medical professionals are a different breed of students who have to have direct interaction with what they are learning to be effective, useful, and practical over time in their medical practice.

My additional thought is to provide solid proven business information that can enable many more doctors to remain in medical practice longer by providing them with knowledge and weapons to fight all the devastating intrusions into their medical practices.

Once they have the weapons and know how to use them, their severe frustrations with what's happening to them and their medical practices will be brought to a minimum because they now know how to defend themselves.

Hopefully, most of the physicians who have reached their maximum tolerance of imputed allegations and professional impeachment by those who make a living by preying on physicians will "stay the course" rather than fall into the desolate list of physician attritions.

Also, and most important of all, most physicians will have the business knowledge to *avoid and prevent the common financial failures* of medical practices we hear about nearly every day.

Why I write articles and books today.

My writing efforts actually began as an afterthought in 1974 at the beginning of my venture into private medical practice, when I became so fed up with the commercial whitewashed patient medical information brochures that weren't worth the paper they were printed on.

When you've experienced witnessing or participating in what happens to the great ideas and projects that are remanufactured by committees, teams, groups, consultants, and prima-donnas, you know how quickly whitewashed these fantastic ideas become. Forgive me for saying this, but dictators have the advantage of never depending on committees.

I created a barrage of medical information and advice on handouts for my patients to read in the 1970s. Medical patients at that time were smart enough to understand issues in medical care. Patients were hungry for medical information that I didn't have time to give them verbally during office hours. Many patients who took the handouts about the various OBG problems and solutions probably never read it all (one or two printed pages), but at least they had the opportunity to do so.

In my medical community, no doctor was doing this for their own medical patients. Thirty years later, I discovered that what I was doing was actually marketing my medical practice without me knowing it at the time. Patients who didn't throw away the handout without reading it would take it home or back to their office where they may read it. When others see a printed handout on a medical topic lying around they pick it up and read it for their own benefit; it was like a free gift and it certainly was a cost-free method of marketing my practice.

I believe that the majority of medical patients really have a desire not only to gather more medical information, but also to know what their own doctor thinks about medical problems when they are sitting there is the exam room with the doctor, and the doctor will rarely take time to talk about.

They'd see my name and address at the end and know that this doctor cared enough for his patients to give them more special information that they would likely never find anywhere else in their lifetime. That kind of doctor draws in new patients.

I later discovered that none of the other physicians in my area were using printed handouts to inform their own patients about medical topics, like I had been doing.

Patients want to read and understand what their own doctor believes and thinks about medical topics... not what those "other doctors" believe. The media often gives out misleading or wrong medical info that confuses patients about who's telling the truth.

However, handout problems for me came from within my own medical community.

I always spent more than usual time talking with my post-op patients before they were discharged from the hospital to give them post-op instructions.

I had learned that after major surgery patients healed faster and with fewer problems and risks when most of the customary post-op restrictions were removed. Restrictions which almost all gyn surgeons had been taught to recommend to their patients seemed far outdated.

The worst time to give your patients specific post-op instructions is the morning they will be discharged. Patients are excited, are in the middle of their preparations to go home, are thinking about what their home situation will be like, and are pretending to listen to their doctor's instructions. That's why printed instructions are great reminders of what their doctor told them.

After taking into account the number of post-op phone calls to my office after my patients (which were few in number) went home because they had already forgotten what I had verbally told them, I decided to print instructions that the patients could take home. So rather than call me, they would read the printed instructions instead. This approach enabled the office to run better without those common post-op patient calls.

I would take a small stack of those post-op instructions and store them in an out-of-the-way spot at the hospital nurse's station on the OB-Gyn floor of the hospital. The day before my patient's discharge, I'd hand my patient the post-op instruction sheet so they had time to read it and could then clear up their questions to me the next morning when they were discharged.

The trouble began when a nurse on the Gyn post-op floor told me that one of my doctor friends told the floor nurses not to put his post-op patients in the same room with mine. It turned out that my patients, at the request of his patients in the same room, would share my post-op instructions with them.

He was a surgeon, for example, who insisted on six weeks of bed rest for his patients after major surgery, contrary to my instructions which told my patients to do anything they wanted whenever they felt ready to do them. I certainly wasn't going to give up what I believed, regardless.

The nurses did their best to put his patients elsewhere, but then the problems escalated to ridiculous levels. Apparently, the word spread among all the OBG doctors, none of whom had printed post-op instructions, about what my patients continued to do: share my post-op instructions with all the patients in the same room who insisted on reading them despite my request to my patients not to share them.

For the next two months, when I arrived to make rounds on my post-op patients, it became necessary to search for where my stack of printed instruction sheets had been moved, retrieve them from the nursing station wastebasket, or find the stack completely gone.

I never was able to discover who was doing all these things to my instruction sheets. But it did paint a bad picture about the professional people I had worked with for many years prior.

Wouldn't that disrespectful activity seem unwarranted and overly aggressive when one considers that I also continued to verbally instruct all my patients at the bedside post-op, where all the other patients of all the other doctors in the patient's room would hear everything I had said to my patient? I even offered to let the other doctors use my instructions, and modify them to fit their own beliefs. No takers!

Was I making enemies and didn't know that I had been… apparently so.

I continued using my same handouts for years to come. In fact, the essence of my post-op instructions came from a wise old general surgeon who also convinced me to follow his advice about patient care post-op. For one thing... to order a regular diet immediately after surgery on my major post-op gyn surgery patients, and did it for all my years in practice without one problem that I can remember... ever!

Allowing patients to eat right after major abdominal or pelvic surgery was the opposite of what we were taught during training. I found that food of any type eaten after surgery stimulated the bowels to work instead of the bowels silently collecting air up until they became obstructed after a few days. Eating prevented the problem—and no other doctor would believe me.

I often wonder how many thousands of patients post-op have had to put up with the usual "NPO" after surgery when it wasn't really necessary.

If there ever was a lesson here, this example should serve as a true indication of how useless it is to try to change the beliefs of any medical professional who developed a stiff-necked mindset for traditional teachings while in medical school and in medical practice. And that goes for traditional medical education scholars as well.

"No matter how great the talents or efforts, some things just take time. You can't produce a baby in one month by getting nine women pregnant."
-Warren Buffett

I continue to write articles for medical patients to read online at www.ezinearticles.com , www.healthcare-toolbox.com, and other article submission sites, and have had several published in Medical Economics, Modern Physician, and on other medical websites. Writing and informing people about medical problems and solutions is something I get great pleasure out of doing.

My rule with writing is to stay far away from fiction as I can, document sources, and provide practical advice and information (the only kind that people will use).

For those who are interested, my updated CV is available online at: www.curtisgrahammd.com

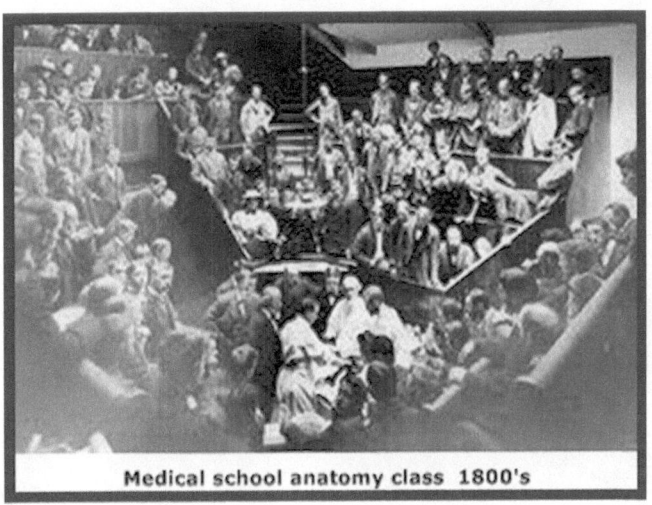

Medical school anatomy class 1800's

Being reminded about what medical education was like in the old days and about the struggles they had teaching medical students without the use of the resources available today, was a remarkable accomplishment.

Providing medical students with an academic business education is no less of an accomplishment.

APPENDIX 1

Evidence Based References – Resources

"Over 114 Highly Recommended_References for a Thorough, Practical Working Knowledge of Business and Marketing for All Physicians and Healthcare Providers"

Business Education – Online Organizations that provide it.

1. National Business Education Association (NBEA)
   National business education standards

2. Higher Education Organizations
   Institute for Higher Education Policies (IHEP)

3. The Journal of Education for Business (J Educ Bus)
   www.researchgate.net

4. List of FREE Online Continuing Education for Business Professionals
   www.education-portal.com

5. COURSERA –FREE courses in business + management
   www.coursera.org

6. Ten Places to get a Free Business Education Online www.education-portal.com

Medical Practice Business Articles... (over 65 of them)

www.marketingamedicalpractice.com/article_archives.htm

Recommended Business Books...

Help For Doctors to Earn More Money an Easier Way than Seeing More Patients and Working Harder.

(References are not listed in any order of preference, educational benefit, or recommended content)

1. **Management: Tasks, Responsibilities, Practices** – Peter F Drucker © 1973-1974, ISBN 0-06-091207-3.

2. **Marketing Your Clinical Practice: Ethically, Effectively, Economically** – Neil Baum, MD, and Gretchen Henkel, © 2004, ISBN-13: 978-0-7637-6983-3, 4th edition.

3. **The Business of Medical Practice: Advanced Profit Maximization Techniques for Savvy Doctors** – David Edward Marcinko, © 2004, ISBN 0-8261-2375-9, 2nd edition.

4. **Medical Practice Management in the 21st Century: The Handbook** – Marjorie A. Satinsky with Randall T. Curnow, Jr., MD, © 2007, ISBN-10 1 84619 023 1.

5. **The New Psycho-Cybernetics:** - Maxwell Maltz, MD (Update by Dan S. Kennedy), © 2001, ISBN 0-7352-0275-3, Revised Edition.

6. **The E-Myth Physician: Why Most Medical Practices Don't Work and What to Do About It** – Michael E. Gerber, © 2003, ISBN 0-06-621469-6.

7. **Getting Everything You Can Out of All you've Got** - Jay Abraham, © 2000, ISBN 0-312-28454-3 (pbk).

8. **No B.S. Ruthless Management of People & Profits** - Dan S. Kennedy, © 2008, ISBN-13: 978-1-59918-165-3.

9. **No B.S. Success in the New Economy** – Dan S. Kennedy, © 2010, ISBN-10: 1-59918-361-7.

10. **No B.S. Trust-Based Marketing** – Dan S. Kennedy and Matt Zagula, © 2012, ISBN-10: 1-59918-440-0.

11. **No B.S. Grassroots Marketing: Local Small Businesses** – Dan S. Kennedy and Jeff Slutsky, © 2012, ISBN-10: 1-59918-439-7.

12. **No B.S. Marketing to Leading Edge Boomers & Seniors** – Dan S. Kennedy and Chip Kessler, © 2013, ISBN-10: 1-59918-450-8.

13. **No B.S. Sales Success** – Dan S. Kennedy, © 2004, ISBN 1-932156-89-5.

14. **No B.S. Price Strategy** – Dan S. Kennedy and Jason Marrs, © 2011, ISBN-10: 1-59918-400-1.

15. **No B.S. Direct Marketing** – Dan S. Kennedy, © 2006, ISBN 1-932531-57-2.

16. **No B.S. Time Management for Entrepreneurs** – Dan S. Kennedy, © 2004, ISBN 1-932156-85-2.

17. **No B.S. Wealth Attraction for Entrepreneurs** – Dan S. Kennedy, © 2006, ISBN 1-932531—67-X.

18. **No B.S. Marketing to the Affluent** – Dan S. Kennedy, © 2008, ISBN-10: 159918-181-9.

19. **No B.S. Business Success** – Dan S. Kennedy, © 2004, ISBN 978-1-932531-10-7.

20. **The Official Get Rich Guide to Information Marketing** – Robert Skrob, © 2011, ISBN-10: 1-59918-410-9.

21. **How to Make Millions With Your Ideas** – Dan S. Kennedy, © 1996, ISBN 0-452-27316-1.

22. **The Ultimate Success Secret** – Dan S. Kennedy, © 2008 Revised edition, Publ. Kennedy Inner Circle, Inc., 5818 N. 7th St. #103, Phoenix, AZ 85014

23. **Make'em Laugh & Take Their Money** – Dan S. Kennedy, © 2010, ISBN 978-0-98237-934-9.

24. **Making Them Believe: 21 Principles** – Dan S. Kennedy and Chip Kessler, © 2010, ISBN: 978-0-98237-938-7.

25. **The Ultimate Marketing Plan** – Dan S. Kennedy, © 2011 4rd Edition, ISBN-10: 1-4405-1184-5.

26. **The Ultimate Sales Letter** – Dan S. Kennedy, © 2006 3rd Edition, ISBN 1-59337-499-2.

27. **The Practice of Management** – Peter F. Drucker, © 1954, ISBN 0-06-091316-9.

28. **My Life in Advertising & Scientific Advertising** – Claude C. Hopkins, © 1966, publ. 1989 by National Textbook Co. 4255 W. Touhy Ave., Lincolnwood, Ill. 60646-1975.

29. **The 22 Immutable Laws of Branding** – Al Ries and Laura Ries, © 2002, ISBN-10: 0-06-000773-7.

30. **Positioning: The Battle for Your Mind** – Al Ries and Jack Trout, © 2001, ISBN 0-07-135916-8.

31. **The New Positioning** – Jack Trout with Steve Rivkin, © 1996, ISBN 0-07-065328-3.

32. **5 Steps to Professional Presence** – Susan Bixler and Lisa Scherrer Dugan, © 2001, ISBN 10: 1-58062-442-1.

33. **The Adweek Copywriting Handbook** – Joseph Sugarman, © 2007, ISBN-10: 0-470-05124-8.

34. **Secrets of Successful Direct Mail** – Richard V. Benson, © 2005 3rd Edit., ISBN 0-88723-334-1.

35. **Influence: The Psychology of Persuasion** – Robert B. Cialdini, PhD, © 1984 Revised Edition, ISBN 0-688-12816-5

36. **Maximum Influence: The 12 Universal Laws of Power Persuasion** – Kurt W. Mortensen, © 2013 2nd Edition, ISBN-10: 0-8144-3209-3.

37. **Confessions of an Advertising Man** – David Ogilvy, © 1987 3rd Edit., ISBN 10: 1-904915-01-9.

38. **Persuasive Online Copywriting** – Bryan Eisenberg, Jeffrey Eisenberg, Lisa T. Davis © 2003, 2nd Edit., ISBN 0-9714769-9-3.

39. **Rich Dad: The Business School** – Robert T. Kiyosaki with Sharon L. Lechter, © 2005 2nd Edit., Publ. Momentum Media, CashFlow Technologies, Inc., 4330 N. Civic Center Plaza, #100, Scottsdale, AZ 85251

40. **Rich Dad: Cashflow Quadrant: Guide to Financial Freedom** – Robert T. Kiyosaki with Sharon L. Lechter, © 1999, ISBN 0-446-67747-7

41. **Rich Dad: Rich Kid Smart Kid** – Robert T. Kiyosaki, © 2012 2nd Edit., ISBN 978-1-61268-060-6.

42. **Rich Dad Poor Dad for Teens** – Robert T. Kiyosaki with Sharon Lechter, © 2004, ISBN 978-0-446-69321-9.

43. **Guerrilla P.R.** – Michael Levine, © 1993 2nd Edit., ISBN 978-0-06-143852-3.

44. **The Million Dollar Total Business Transformation** – Walter Bergeron, © 2012, ISBN 978-1477401354.

45. **The Art and Science of Success (Vol. 2)** – Matt Morris + co-authors, © 2011, ISBN 978-0-9830770-1-5.

46. **Great Legal Marketing** – Benjamin W. Glass, III, © 2012, ISBN 978-0-98371-251-0.

47. **Success Is an Inside Job** – Lee Milteer, © 2005, ISBN 1-57174-1194.

48. **Yes: 50 Scientifically Proven Ways to Be Persuasive** – Robert B. Cialdini, Noah Goldstein, Steve Martin - © 2008, ISBN-10: 1-4165-7096-9.

49. **The 12 Factors of Business Success** – Kevin Hogan, Dave Lakhani, Mollie Marti, © 2008, ISBN 978-0-470-29299-0.

50. **Global Brand Power** – Barbara E. Kahn, © 2013, Wharton School of Business, ISBN 978-1-61363-025-9.

51. **Customer Centricity** – Peter Fader, © 2012, Wharton School of Business, ISBN 978-1-61363-016-7.

52. **The Direct Mail Solution** – Craig Simpson with Dan S. Kennedy, © 2014, ISBN-10: 1-59918-518-0.

53. **Smart Medicine** – William Hanson, MD, © 2011, ISBN 978-0-230-62115-2.

54. **Consumer Satisfaction in Medical Practice** – Paul A. Sommers, PhD, © 1999, ISBN 0-7890-0713-4

55. **The New Medical Marketplace** – Anne Stoline, MD, and Jonathan P. Weiner, PhD, © 1988, ISBN 0-8018-3645-X

56. **Start Your Own Medical Practice** – Judge William Huss and Marlene M. Coleman, MD**,** © 2006, ISBN-13: 978-1-57248-574-7.

57. **The Medical Entrepreneur: Pearls, Pitfalls & Practical Business Advice For Doctors** –Steven M. Hacker, MD, © 2010, ISBN-10: 0615407137.

58. **Spiritual Power Tools: For Successful Selling** – Lee Milteer, © 2005, ISBN 1-57174-428-2.

59. **Tested Advertising Methods** – John Caples (Revised by Fred E. Hahn), © 1997 5th Edition, ISBN 0-13-244609-X ISBN 0-13-095701-1.

60. **Differentiate or Die** – Jack Trout with Steve Rivkin, © 2000, ISBN 0-471-35764-2.

61. **Marketing Strategies for the Home Based Business** – Shirley George Frazier, © 2008, ISBN-13: 978-0-7627-4240-0.

62. **The Robert Collier Letter Book** – Robert Collier, © 1937, ISBN 0-912576-21-9.

63. **Selling: Powerful New Strategies for Sales Success** – Kevin Hogan, Dave Lakhani, Gary May Mollie Marti, Eliot Hoppe, Larry Adams, © 2008, ISBN 978-1-934266-04-5.

64. **101 Ways to Promote Yourself** – Raleigh Pinskey, © 1997, ISBN 0-380-81054-9.

65. **The Irresistible Offer: How to sell your service in 3 seconds of less** – Mark Joyner, © 2005, ISBN-10: 0-471-73894-8.

66. **Triggers: 30 sales tools to motivate, influence, persuade** – Joseph Sugarman, © 1999, ISBN 1-891686-03-8.

67. **The Science of Influence** – Kevin Hogan, © 2005, ISBN 0-471-67051-0.

68. **Power and Persuasion: How to command success in business** – Michael Masterson, © 2005, ISBN-13: 978-0-471-7-86771.

69. **How to Persuade People Who Don't Want to be Persuaded** – Joel Bauer and Mark Levy, © 2004, ISBN 0-471-64797-7.

70. **Secrets of Online Persuasion** – John-Paul and Deborah Micek, © 2006, ISBN 1-60037-029-2.

71. **The Laws of Charisma** – Kurt W. Mortensen, © 2011, ISBN-10: 0-8144-1591-1.

72. **Mind Capture** – Tony Rubleski, © 2008, ISBN 978-1-60037-457-9.

73. **Never Be Lied To Again** – David J. Lieberman, PhD, © 1998, ISBN 0-312-18634-7.

74. **How To Change Anybody** – David J. Lieberman, PhD, © 2005, ISBN 0-312-32474-X.

75. **Threshold Resistance** – A. Alfred Taubman, © 2007, ISBN 978-0-06-123537-5.

76. **How To Be A Great Communicator** – Nido R. Qubein, © 1997, ISBN 0-471-16314-7.

77. **Top Performance: Develop Excellence in Yourself and Others** – Zig Ziglar, © 2003 Revised and Updated 2005, ISBN 0-8007-1828-3.

78. **Using Psychology: Principles of Behavior and Your Life** – Morris K. Holland, © 1975, Library of Congress Catalog Card NO. 74-25502

79. **Get Anyone To Do Anything: Never feel powerless again** – David J. Lieberman, PhD, © 2000, ISBN 0-312-20904-5.

80. **Prosper** – Ethan Willis and Randy Garn, © 2011, ISBN 978-1-60994-070-6.

81. **The Magic Power of Emotional Appeal** – Roy Garn, © 1960, Libr. Congress # 60-10848.

82. **Covert Persuasion** – Kevin Hogan and James Speakman, © 2006, ISBN-10: 0-470-05141-8.

83. **Subliminal Persuasion: Influence and Marketing Secrets** – Dave Lakhani, © 2008, ISBN 978-0-470-24336-7.

84. **Persuasion: The Art of Getting What You Want** – Dave Lakhani, © 2005, ISBN-10: 0-471-73044-0.

85. **Sell Your Brain Power** – Fred Gleeck, © 2012, ISBN 978-0-936965-99-4.

86. **Marketing to The Affluent** – Dr. Thomas J. Stanley, PhD, © 1988, ISBN 0-07-061047-9.

87. **The Ultimate Sales Machine: Turbocharge Your Business, 12 Key Strategies** – Chet Holmes, © 2007, ISBN 978-1-59184-160-9.

88. **The Long Tail: Future of Business** – Chris Anderson, © 2006, ISBN 1-4013-0237-8.

89. **Call To Action** – Bryan Eisenberg and Jeffrey Eisenberg, © 2005, ISBN 1-932226-39-7.

90. **Advertising Secrets of The Written Word** – Joseph Sugarman, © 1998, ISBN 1-891686-00-3.

91. **Ultimate Small Business Marketing Guide** – James Stephenson, © 2003, ISBN 1-932156-10-0.

92. **How To Write A Good Advertisement: Short Course in Copywriting** – Victor O. Schwab, © 1962, ISBN 0-87980-397-7.

93. **Ogilvy On Advertising** – David Ogilvy, © 1983, ISBN 0-517-55075-X.

94. **Straight Talk About Small Business** – Kenneth J. Albert, © 1981, ISBN 0-07-000949-X.

95. **First Impressions** – Ann Demarais, PhD, and Valerie White, PhD., © 2004, ISBN 0-553-38201-2.

96. **The Entrepreneur's Secret To Creating Wealth: How the Smartest Business Owners Build Their Fortunes** – Chris Hurn, © 2012, ISBN 978-1-59932-315-2.

97. **The Charge: Activating 10 Human Drives** – Brendon Burchard, © 2012, ISBN 978-1-4516-6753-0.

98. **Reading People: Understand people and predict their behavior** – Jo-Ellan Dimitrius, PhD, and Mark Mazzarella, © 1998, ISBN 0-375-50146-0.

99. **Ready, Fire, Aim: Zero to 100 Million in No Time Flat** – Michael Masterson, © 2008, ISBN 978-0-470-18202-4.

100. **OPM: Other People's Money: How to attract OPM** – Michael A. Lechter, Esq., © 2005, ISBN 0-446-69185-2.

101. **The 22 Immutable Laws of Marketing** – Al Ries and Jack Trout, © 1993, ISBN 0-88730-592-X.

102. **Hire Your First Employee** – Rhonda Abrams, © 2010, ISBN 978-1-933895-15-4.

103. **Guerrilla Marketing for Consultants** – Jay Conrad Levinson and Michael W. McLaughlin, © 2005, ISBN 0-471-61873-X.

104. **Marketing Warfare** – Al Ries and Jack Trout, © 2006, ISBN 0-07-146082-9.

105. **Uncensored Sales Strategies** – Sydney Biddle Barrows with Dan S. Kennedy, © 2009, ISBN-10: 1-59918-193-2.

106. **The Mastermind Marketing System** – Jay Abraham, Nightingale-Conant, www.nightinggale.com Money Making Power Principles for Your Business Success.

107. **Think and Grow Rich** – by Napoleon Hill, © 1937, 17 business principles for successful business ventures.

108. **SK&A (A Cegedim Company)** – www.skainfo.com – Medical profession data products, data services, data optimization – Healthcare research reports.

109. **Financial Peace** – By Dave Ramsey

APPENDIX 2

Core Foundations

"Foundational Medical Practice Responsibilities of Physicians and Healthcare Providers"

What the Hippocratic Oath Really Says...

THE COMMONLY QUOTED and referred to phrase, **"First, do no harm," has *never been part of the Hippocratic Oath.*** The derivation of that phrase came from Hippocrates' *"Epidemics."* He wrote, *"Declare the past, diagnose the present, foretell the future; practice these acts. As to diseases, make a habit of two things—to help, or* **at least to do no harm.***"*

Hippocrates thoughts about the ten commandments
(Source: Wikipedia authors and information)

The oath Hippocrates wrote was not meant to be a moral guide for anyone but physicians. Anyone who reads the "real" original version sees it was an effort by Hippocrates to create a standard for acceptable practice of medicine by doctors.

The oath was written to meet the "beliefs of that day." Christianity didn't spring up for four hundred more years. Hippocrates must have thought about to some degree the need to keep revising the oath to match the changing morals and beliefs over the years. Clinging to outdated dogma is a function of misguided intelligence.

Consider first one of the most accurate translations of the original Greek document.

Original version…

I swear by Apollo the healer, Aesculapius, Health/all the powers of healing, and call to witness all the gods/goddesses that I may keep this Oath/Promise to the best of my ability/judgment.

I will *pay the same respect to my master in the Science as to my parents/share my life with him/pay all my debts to him.*

… regard his sons as my brothers/teach them the Science, if they desire to learn it, without fee/contract.

… hand on precepts, lectures, all other learning to my sons, to those of my master, to those pupils duly apprenticed/sworn, and to none other.

… use my power to help the sick to the best of my ability/judgment; I will abstain from harming/wronging any man by it.

… not give a fatal draught to anyone if I am asked nor suggest any such thing. Neither will I give a woman means to procure an abortion.

… be chaste/religious in my life/in my practice.

… not cut, even for the stone, but I will leave such procedures to the practitioners of that craft. Whenever I go into a house, I will go to help the sick/never with the intention of doing harm/injury.

… not abuse my position to indulge in sexual contacts with the bodies of women/men, whether they be freemen/slaves. Whatever I see or hear, professionally/privately, which ought not to be divulged, I will keep secret/tell no one.

If I observe this Oath/do not violate it, may I prosper both in my life/in my profession, earning good repute among all men for my time. If I transgress/forswear this oath, may my lot be otherwise.

(Abbreviated for editorial compliance)

(Translated by J. Chadwick and W. N. Mann, 1950)

Adaptation of the oath…

Many updated versions of the oath have been made. The second major change of the oath was in 1943. Most of the changes have been made in the last century. The rapidly expanding expertise, knowledge, and research are the reasons. To make the oath more understandable and yet keep it in the Greek and Roman style of simplicity and form, the classical version was born.

Classical version…

I swear by Apollo Physician/Asclepius/Hygieia/Panaceia/the gods/goddesses, making them witnesses, I will fulfill according to my ability/judgment this oath/ covenant:

To hold him who taught me this art equal to my parents/to live my life in partnership with him, if he is in need of money, give him a share of mine, regard his offspring equal to my brothers in male lineage, teach them this art-if they desire to learn—without fee/covenant; give a share of precepts/oral instruction/the other learning to my sons, the sons of him who instructed me, pupils who have signed the covenant, have taken an oath according to the medical law, but no one else.

I will apply dietetic measures for benefit of the sick according to my ability/judgment; keep them from harm/injustice.

I will neither give a deadly drug to anybody who asked for it, nor make a suggestion to this effect. Similarly, not give to a woman an abortive remedy.

In purity/holiness I will guard my life/art.

I will not use the knife, not on sufferers from stone, but withdraw in favor of such men as are engaged in this work.

Whatever houses I visit, I come for the benefit of the sick, remaining free of intentional injustice, mischief, in particular sexual relations with both female/male persons, be they free/slaves.

What I see/hear in the course of the treatment, even outside treatment in regard to life of men, which on no account must spread abroad, I will keep to myself, holding such things shameful to be spoken about.

If I fulfill this oath, not violate it, may it be granted me to enjoy life/art, being honored with fame among men for time to come; if I transgress, swear falsely, may the opposite of this be my lot.

(Abbreviated for editorial compliance)

From The Hippocratic Oath: Text, Translation, and Interpretation, *by Ludwig Edelstein. Baltimore: Johns Hopkins Press, 1943.*

Modern implications and relevance…

Although the Oath is widely believed to have been written by Hippocrates or even a student of his, some are proposing that Pythagoreans might have written it. Modern-day views of the Oath are considered primarily of historical or traditional value.

Examining the traditional modern-day text of the oath makes it even more understandable—not necessarily more appropriate for 2014. The Hippocratic Oath has been rewritten to match the ethics and conduct of doctors many times especially in the past century.

That's understandable because the specifics of the oath are outdated relative to professional and societal changes that have been rapidly changing over the last one hundred years. The traditional text of the oath is an effort to make it more understandable. The more conversational text does not remove any of the original document or meaning.

Traditional text of the oath...

I swear by Apollo the physician, by Aesculapius, Hygeia, and Panacea, and I take to witness all the gods, all the goddesses, to keep according to my ability and my judgment, the following oath.

"To consider dear to me as my parents him who taught me this art; to live in common with him and if necessary to share my goods with him; to look upon his children as my own brothers, to teach them this art if they so desire without fee or written promise; to impart to my sons and the sons of the master who taught me and the disciples who have enrolled themselves and have agreed to the rules of the profession, but to these alone the precepts and the instruction.

I will prescribe regimens for the good of my patients according to my ability and my judgment and never do harm to anyone. To please no one will I prescribe a deadly drug nor give advice, which may cause his death.

Nor will I give a woman a pessary to procure abortion.
I will not cut for stone. I will leave this operation to be performed by practitioners, specialists in this art.

In every house where I come I will enter only for the good of my patients, keeping myself far from all intentional ill-doing and all seduction and especially from the pleasures of love with women or with men, be they free or slaves.

All that may come to my knowledge in the exercise of my ought not to be spread abroad, I will keep secret and will never reveal.

If I keep this oath faithfully, may I enjoy my life and practice my art,; but if I swerve from it or violate it, may the reverse be my lot."

(Edited, shortened to meet editorial compliance)

Shall we dump the Hippocratic Oath—or make a new oath?

Who wants to make an oath to pagan gods? Major revisions on the Oath will permit it to remain an acceptable tradition of our academic medical system. Revisions would have to be so drastic that a new oath would be a better choice. If that were done, then what would the plaintiff malpractice attorneys have left to present to the jury?

The problems with the old Oath are very obvious. It promoted men as physicians only. Primary care doctors could not do surgery, which is far from the truth today. Abortion was forbidden. Doctors weren't allowed to participate in assisted suicide situations.

The Oath from about 400 BC did not cover such controversial issues as in vitro fertilization, contraception use, morning-after pills, living wills, health management organizations, and government-mandated medical care.

These issues could be added to the old oath in the form of amendments—like our Constitution has. But the process would never be as effective as that of creating a new formal oath and revised as necessary to keep up with the times.

Substitute Oaths have been used by medical schools…

During the 1970s, many American medical schools were faced with the "oath dilemma." Social and cultural influences made it prudent for medical schools to abandon the Hippocratic Oath as part of the graduating ceremonies. The oath or prayer of Maimonides was substituted.

The oath came under scrutiny by doctors and others in the 1970s with the rise of political correctness and relevance issues. Any oath must be pertinent, accurate, and conform to society pressures. The Hippocratic Oath didn't.

Maimonides clearly understood a physician's obligations to patients, the necessity of updating medical knowledge, and compassion for the sick.

The Oath of Maimonides...

"The eternal providence has appointed me to watch over the life and health of Thy creatures. May the love for my art actuate me at all time; may neither avarice nor miserliness, nor thirst for glory or for a great reputation engage my mind; for the enemies of truth and philanthropy could easily deceive me and make me forgetful of my lofty aim of doing good to Thy children.

May I never see in the patient anything but a fellow creature in pain.

Grant me the strength, time and opportunity always to correct what I have acquired, always to extend its domain; for knowledge is immense and the spirit of man can extend indefinitely to enrich itself daily with new requirements.

Today he can discover his errors of yesterday and tomorrow he can obtain a new light on what he thinks himself sure of today. Oh, God, Thou hast appointed me to watch over the life and death of Thy creatures; here am I ready for my vocation and now I turn unto my calling."

Bio: Moses Maimonides (1135/38-1204) (in Hebrew: Rav or Rabbi Moshe Ben Maimon or "RaMBaM" – the acronym of his name) was the most important Jewish philosopher of the middle ages. Maimonides was born in the Spanish city of Cordoba at a time when about one-fifth of the people in southern Spain were Jews. However, Maimonides and his family fled to Fustat (now Cairo) because of rising anti-Semitism in Spain. There Maimonides worked as a physician, but also became a scholar of Jewish law and a philosopher.

The "Daily Prayer of a Physician" is attributed to Maimonides, but was probably written by Marcus Herz, a German physician, pupil of Immanuel Kant, and physician to Moses Mendelssohn. It first appeared in print in about 1793. (Source: Wikipedia authors and information)

The Prayer of Maimonides...

"Almighty God, Thou hast created human body with infinite wisdom. Ten thousand times ten thousand organs hast Thou combined that act unceasingly, harmoniously to preserve the whole body.

Thou endowed man with wisdom to relieve suffering of his brother, recognize his disorders, extract healing substances, discover their powers prepare and apply them to suit every ill.

Do not allow thirst for profit, ambition for renown and admiration, to interfere with my profession. Illumine my mind that it recognize what presents itself, that it may comprehend what is absent, hidden. Let it not fail to see what is visible, Let me never be absentminded.

May no strange thoughts divert my attention at the bedside of the sick, disturb my mind in its silent labors, for great, sacred are the thoughtful deliberations required to preserve lives, health of Thy creatures.

Grant that my patients have confidence in me, my art, follow my directions, counsel. Remove from their midst charlatans, host of officious relatives, know-all nurses, cruel people who arrogantly frustrate wisest purposes of our art, often lead Thy creatures to their death.

Should those who are wiser than I wish to improve and instruct me, let my soul gratefully follow their guidance. Should conceited fools, censure me, I remain steadfast without regard for age, reputation, honor.

Imbue my soul with gentleness and calmness when older colleagues, wish to displace me, scorn me, to teach me.

Never allow the thought to arise in me that I have attained sufficient knowledge, but ever to extend my knowledge. For art is great, but the mind of man is ever expanding.

I now apply myself to my profession. Support me in this great task so that it may benefit mankind, for without Thy help not even the least thing will succeed."

(Edited, shortened, to meet editorial compliance)

(Translated by Harry Friedenwald) *Bulletin of the Johns Hopkins Hospital*
28: 260-261, (1917)

Wikipedia and what today conflicts with the Oath:

Wikipedia, the free encyclopedia, while acknowledging the Hippocratic Oath as a traditional value, goes on to list ten separate issues mentioned in the oath that *are in direct conflict with modern-day medical care and physician conduct.*

1. ***To teach medicine to the sons of my teacher***. In the past, medical schools would give preferential consideration to the children of physicians. This too has largely disappeared.

2. ***Not to teach medicine to other people.*** A physician who has a hand in half-educating quacks or other people not enrolled in an approved medical school would likely lose his or her license even today.

3. ***To practice and prescribe to the best of my ability for the good of my patients and to try to avoid harming them.*** This beneficial intention is the purpose of the physician. However, this item is still invoked in discussions of euthanasia.

4. ***To never deliberately do harm to anyone for anyone else's interest.*** Physician organizations in the United States and most other countries have strongly denounced physician participation in legal executions.

5. ***To never attempt to induce an abortion.*** The wide availability of abortions in much of the world suggests that many physicians no longer feel bound by this.

6. ***To avoid violating the morals of my community.*** Many licensing agencies will revoke a physician's license for offending the morals of the community ("moral turpitude").

7. ***To avoid attempting to do things that other specialists can do better.*** The "stones" referred to are kidney stones or bladder stones, removal of which was judged too difficult for physicians, and therefore was left for surgeons (specialists). It is interesting how early the value of specialization was recognized. The range of knowledge and skills needed for the range of human problems has always made it impossible for any single physician to maintain expertise in all areas.

8. ***To keep the good of the patient as the highest priority.*** There may be other conflicting "good purposes," such as community welfare, conserving economic resources, supporting the criminal justice system, or simply making money for the physician or his employer that provide recurring challenges to physicians.

9. ***To avoid sexual relationships or other inappropriate entanglements with patients and families.*** The value of avoiding conflicts of interest has never been questioned.

10. ***To keep confidential all private patient information.*** Confidentiality between physician and patient continues to be valued and protected, but governments and third-parties have occasionally encroached upon it.

What is it that hinders the task of bringing the Hippocratic Oath back into relevance again?

1. Can one oath apply to all doctors? With the division of medicine into specialties comes a separation of focus, commitment, and ethics to a degree. So how is it possible to include all those differences into one code or oath?

2. How do you create a core of moral values that are acceptable to every religion or religious belief?

3. Should there be a separate oath for each division of medical practice? A doctor who participates in "assisted suicide" has a completely different set of ethics than one who abhors the same issue.

4. Should the Oath be a very generalized expression of superficial and almost meaningless value that fits everybody? In that case, why even have an oath?

5. Since the Hippocratic Oath was originally cast in a mold of pagan idealism, is it just better to create a new Oath instead of revising the original one?

6. Is it even possible to create an oath that goes beyond cheap formality and reaches a level of being a binding covenant of conduct and ethics that all doctors will abide by?

7. Should it be in the form of a "creed" or "credo," which is any system of codification of any belief or opinion? Should it be in form of an "oath," which is a formally affirmed statement, or series of statements, accompanied by a promise?

8. Is a "vow" or "pledge" a way to avoid the bad word "oath?" Being a solemn earnest promise and personal commitment to professional accountability, a vow might take on the ambiance of the more acceptable and assertive promise. A pledge might even be better because of its agreement to abide by an issue with the idea that it assumes there is an exchange of one thing for another. If one pledges, he has not been fully accepted into that profession.

9. Should a second oath be constructed for the young doctor dissenters who don't believe in any oath. They show disrespect for even the modern version of the Hippocratic Oath and ridicule the medical schools that still revere any oath.

10. Should the new oath be long or short? Including all of the important components of physician conduct presently, as well as most of the ethical issues facing doctors today, would be a long oath. With a short oath both these angles could be condensed into a few weak paragraphs that would negate its credibility.

11. Might one create an oath that adds dignity to the services any doctor performs in his career and forget about the rules of conduct, or the recital of medical ethics? In that case, the medical conduct of doctors as well as the ethical practice issues can be the responsibility of the various specialty groups or national medical organizations. Each would have their own.

12. How should an oath be administered in the medical profession? If you just think it, no one will know whether you believe in the oath or not.

    When you say an oath aloud, it takes on a whole different meaning.

    Speaking the oath makes you accountable to the witnesses. If you sign it, you validate its value to you in front of everyone.

13. What is the purpose of having a medical oath? Besides making a formal and traditional agreement or promise, other values are inherent. By giving an oath, one's mind and heart join in

that promise. The unconscious acceptance of the centuries-old traditions of the medical profession is fixed in the brain.

A subconscious thankfulness for all those who have gone before you for allowing you to share their knowledge and skills is easily overlooked as a purpose for an oath.

And the conscious thoughts of what you can do in the future for the health and welfare of mankind (no longer is a pipedream), that confidence trails along for days or a lifetime after the oath is spoken.

Ouch! That's heavy stuff!

Let's Get Real Here...

What was once the epitome of conduct for the physician (Hippocratic Oath) no longer bears a good resemblance to what is thought today to be good conduct of a physician.

The 1993 survey* of 150 U.S. and Canadian medical schools seems to bury it for good. Of all the various oaths taken by graduates only 14 percent outlaw euthanasia, 8 percent object to abortion, 3 percent forbid sexual contact with patients, 11 percent include a deity mention, and fewer than 50 percent insist that the taker should be held accountable for keeping the oath.

When one takes the time to look deeper into the developing (and perhaps is already here) chasm between the qualities of doctors who were trained before 1960-1965 and the qualities of doctors since, I am personally disappointed by what I see.

The keys to the tight-knit doctor world of sub 1965 have been eroded by a tidal wave of intellectual and spiritual depravation. Does anyone believe in God anymore? Those doctors who really care about conduct, ethics, and morals have made great efforts to demonstrate to the younger doctors the values that count in the medical profession. The best example of that is the modern version of the Hippocratic Oath written by Louis Lasagna, M.D., in 1964. (Source: Wikipedia authors and information)

Below is the version of the oath you need to slap on your wall!

Hippocratic Oath—Modern Version…

I swear to fulfill, to best of my ability, judgment, this covenant:

I will respect hard-won scientific gains of physicians in whose steps I walk, share such knowledge as is mine with those who follow.

… apply, for benefit of sick, all measures required, avoiding those traps of over treatment and therapeutic nihilism.

… remember that there is art to medicine as well as science, that warmth, sympathy, understanding may outweigh the surgeon's knife, chemist's drug.

… not be ashamed to say "I know not," nor will I fail to call in my colleagues when the skills of another are needed for a patient's recovery.

… respect the privacy of my patients, their problems are not disclosed to me that the world may know.

I must tread with care in matters of life and death. But it may also be within my power to take a life; this awesome responsibility must be faced with great humbleness, awareness of my frailty.

… remember that I do not treat a fever chart, a cancerous growth, but a sick human being, whose illness may affect the person's family and economic stability. My responsibility includes these related problems, if I am to care adequately for the sick.

… prevent disease whenever I can, for prevention is preferable to cure.

… remember that I remain a member of society, with special obligations to my fellow human beings, those sound of mind, body as well as the infirm.

If I do not violate this oath, may I enjoy life and art, respected while I live and remembered with affection thereafter. May I always act so as to preserve the finest traditions of my calling and may I long experience the joy of healing those who seek my help.

(Edited, shortened to meet editorial compliance)

(Written in 1964 by Louis Lasagna, Academic Dean of the School of Medicine at Tufts University, and used in many medical schools today.)

There you have it—almost.

The modern version of the oath encompasses most if not all of the vows contained in the original Hippocratic Oath. It has been updated to a level where it is appropriate for modern medical care and rephrases the proper conduct of a physician to match the modern doctor and the cultural mandates he practices by.

It's logical and traditional to have an oath for such a responsible and accountable profession. But then, the "new-generation" doctor is unable to comprehend the value or extent of obligations, commitments, and honor of old. They have become a generation of doctors who are defensive (and rightly so) and cosmopolitan. Who needs an oath?

"Tradition is like a river. It continues to flow and change direction until it reaches it lowest level. But its source core and value always remains at the higher level of its origin."
-C. Graham

The one great aspect of the medical profession that stands out above all others is servant-hood. Ruth Smeltzer describes servant-hood so well:

"You have not lived a perfect day, even though you have earned your money, unless you have done something for someone who will never be able to repay you."
---Ruth Smeltzer

****

American Medical Association (AMA)
(Modern adaptation of the Hippocratic Oath)

THE MODERN OATH OF HIPPOCRATES

(Please read the "Physicians' Charter," a new Charter on medical professionalism.)

That you will be loyal to the Profession of Medicine and just and generous to its members.

That you will lead your lives and practice your art in uprightness and honor.

That into whatsoever house you shall enter, it shall be for the good of the sick to the utmost of your power, you're holding yourselves far aloof from wrong, from corruption, from the tempting of others to vice.

That you will exercise your art solely for the cure of your patients, and will give no drug, perform no operation, for a criminal purpose, even if solicited, far less suggest it.

That whatsoever you shall see or hear of the lives of men or women which is not fitting to be spoken, you will keep inviolably secret.

These things do you swear. Let each bow the head in sign of acquiescence. And now, if you will be true to this, your oath, may prosperity and good repute be ever yours; the opposite, if you shall prove yourselves forsworn.

By Orr, R. D., N. Pang, E. D. Pellegrino, and M. Siegler. 1997. Use of the Hippocratic Oath: A Review of Twentieth Century Practice and a Content Analysis of Oaths Administered in Medical Schools in the U.S. and Canada in 1993. *The Journal of Clinical Ethics* 8 (winter): 377-388.

Addendum: History of the oath...

DECLARATION OF GENEVA.

It is of interest to note that after the Second World War, the *Nuremberg Code of Ethics in Medical Research* was framed to guide the Allied Military Tribunal in the prosecution of Nazi physicians accused of brutal experiments on political prisoners.

As a result, the World Medical Association appointed a committee to prepare a *Charter of Medicine* and to make necessary revisions to bring the *Hippocratic Oath* up to date. Minor changes and substitutions were made in the oath, and in 1948, in Geneva; the Second General Assembly adopted what is now known as *the Declaration of Geneva.*

DECLARATION OF GENEVA

(Adopted by the General Assembly of the World Medical Association at Geneva, Switzerland, September 1948. Given at the time of being admitted as a Member of the Medical Profession)

I SOLEMNLY PLEDGE myself to consecrate my life to the service of humanity.

I WILL GIVE to my teachers the respect and gratitude which is their due.

I WILL PRACTICE my profession with conscience and dignity; THE HEALTH OF MY PATIENT will be my first consideration;

I WILL RESPECT the secrets which are confided in me.

I WILL MAINTAIN by all the means in my power, the honor and the noble traditions of the medical profession; MY COLLEAGUES will be my brothers.

I WILL NOT PERMIT considerations of religion, nationality, race, party politics or social standing to intervene between my duty and my patient.

I WILL MAINTAIN the utmost respect for human life, from the time of conception; even under threat, I will not use my medical knowledge contrary to the laws of humanity.

I MAKE THESE PROMISES solemnly, freely and upon my honor.

Hippocratic Oath References

http://www.pbs.org/wgbh/nova/doctors/oath_modern.html
http://www.pbs.org/wgbh/nova/doctors/oath_classical.html
http://www.indiana.edu/~ancmed/oath.htm
http://classics.mit.edu/Hippocrates/hippooath.html
http://en.wikipedia.org/wiki/Hippocratic_Oath
http://www.geocities.com/everwild7/noharm.html
http://www.bbc.co.uk/dna/h2g2/A1103798
http://www.nlm.nih.gov/hmd/greek/greek_oath.html
http://www.medword.com/hippocrates.html
http://www.answers.com/topic/hippocratic-oath
http://www.annals.org/cgi/content/abstract/138/8/673
http://drblayney.com/Asclepius.html
http://www.answers.com/topic/hippocrates

An Epiphany of Medical Tradition:

Medical caduceus:

If tradition and history means anything to the medical profession, then honoring the profession with a distinguishing symbol that indicates the known roots of the profession would be laudable. Otherwise, the medical profession continues to be further commoditized and irrationally linked to mysticism.

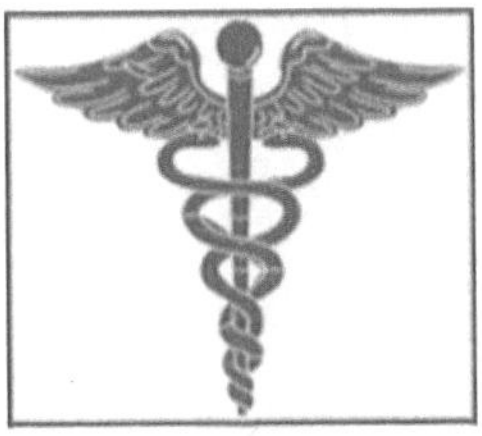

Have you ever wondered why and how this medical symbol came to be accepted in our society in spite of the **double** serpent and **wings** that conflict with the history of traditional medicine and has never been officially supported or adopted as the official insignia of the *practice of medicine*?

This generic symbol/icon standing today for "everything" related to health and medicine, should be redesigned specifically for the medical profession itself, to be consistent with the historically documented medical truth of one snake and no wings.

REFERENCE: The Latin word cādūceus is an adaptation of the Greek κηρύκειον kērukeion, meaning "herald's wand (or staff)", deriving from κῆρυξ kērux, meaning "messenger, herald, envoy". Liddell and Scott, Greek-English Lexicon; Stuart L. Tyson, "The Caduceus", The Scientific Monthly, 34.6, (1932: 492–98) p. 493

Likely copied from:

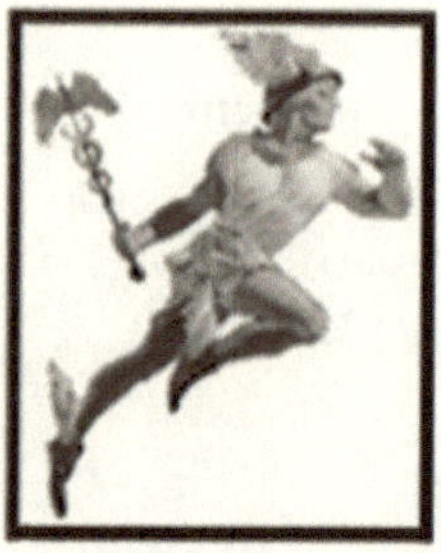

Hermes is a Greek god, fast and crafty, moves in and out of the mortal and divine worlds, messenger, intercessor between mortals and gods, conductor of souls into the afterlife, protector and patron of travelers, herdsmen, thieves, orators and wit, literature and poets, athletics and sports, invention and trade, devises self-satisfaction or for the sake of humankind. **(nothing pertaining to the medical profession)**

His attributes and symbols include the herma, the rooster and the tortoise, purse or pouch, winged sandals, winged cap, and his main symbol is the **herald's staff**, the Greek *kerykeion* or Latin *caduceus* which consisted of two snakes wrapped around a winged staff. (Wikipedia description)

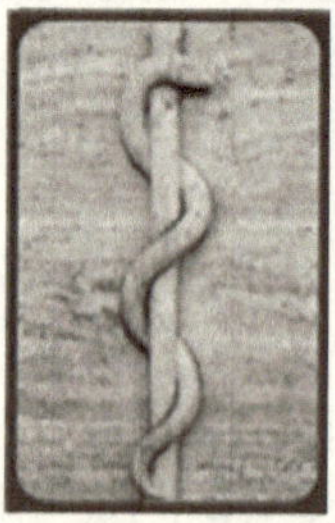

All historical medical profession records, for example, show a staff with only one serpent wound around it, which should be the appropriate symbol of the medical profession. The reasons for this design can be associated directly to the historical records of medical treatment in ancient times.

APPENDIX 3

Healthcare Research

"SK&A – Healthcare Market Research Reports and Services"

THIS ONLINE COMPANY website is a unique healthcare and physician-focused website well worth any physician's use. The constantly updated medical practice information warehouse has no close competitor when it comes to anyone or any medical institution needing to make serious medical practice-related decisions.

The AMA is also a good source of medical practice information and reliable data, but encompasses a much narrower range of attention primarily to physician benefits rather than to the wider medical profession community.

SK&A captures and publishes some of the AMA data, information, and surveys in addition to a widespread number of other companies who do research and publish practical medical information and surveys that I find very useful for physician decision making, especially for private medical practice decisions.

Other very helpful services SK&A provides is free access to physicians for downloading many of the survey and marketing reports as well as job information, medical industry forums, and marketing mailing lists of many kinds.

Physicians can easily use SK&A lists to use in direct mail marketing filtered to a doctor's local community to recruit new medical patients. They create a list specifically targeting the type of patients you want in your practice, their income ranges, their emails, their addresses and phone numbers. They will create mailing lists for you to market to other doctors who might refer you new patients or use you as their doctor consultant for their patients, among others.

One of the most important resources for medical students and other young doctors is their research data on salary compensation levels for twenty-one specialties.

You can go to their website, register for free reports, and download the "U.S. Physician Compensation Trends (Revised 2013)" to begin your search on the average salary (highest and lowest) you can use as a predictable income for your specialty and method of medical practice.

Where else can you find such highly reliable and important information so critical to your medical career decision making?

My pleasure comes from helping you to make a difference in the world of medicine. It might serve you well by visiting these Bible related business inspirations…

Ecclesiastes 3:22-7:12-10:19
Ephesians 4:1
Isaiah 48:17
Deuteronomy 8:18
James 5:12
1 Timothy 6:10
Proverbs 1:5-3:13-4:7-8:11-9:9-10:4-10:15-13:11-16:16-17:27-18:15-19:20-22:29

APPENDIX 4

Physician Compensation Trends

SK&A—Healthcare Market Research Reports

U.S. Physician Compensation Trends

(Revised 2013)

Salary Guidelines	Anesthesiologists	Cardiac & Thoracic Surgeons	Cardiologists
Median salary (1)	$377,375	$544,087	$430,316
Median work RVUs(1)	-	9,500	6.934
Median gross charges (1)	$1,268,671	$1,735,543	$1,400,210
Mean salary for men (2)	$347,000	-	$362,000
Mean salary for women (2)	$300,000	_	$310,000
Highest-paying region (2)	North Central ($383,000)	_	North West ($403,000)
Lowest-paying region (2)	West ($318,000)	-	North East ($311,000)
Hospital-employed salary (2)	$349,000	-	$314,000

Multispecialty group practice salary (2)	$374,000	–	$380,000
Highest offered base salary (3)	$475,000	.	$600,000
Lowest offered base salary (3)	$290,000	-	$275,000
SK&A count of physicians (4)	32,604	4,627	36,510

Salary Guidelines	Dermatology	Diagnostic Radiologists	Emergency Medicine
Median salary (1)	$397,370	$485,277	$297,500
Median work RVUs(1)	7,282	7,813	7,073
Median gross charges (1)	$1,459,936	$2,162,671	$966,814
Mean salary for men (2)	$321,000	-	$183,000
Mean salary for women (2)	$284,000	-	$172,000
Highest-paying region (2)	Great Lakes ($333,000)	-	North East ($228,000)
Lowest-paying region (2)	South Central ($274.000)	-	Northeast ($148,000)
Hospital-employed salary (2)	$117,000	-	$146,000
Multispecialty group practice salary (2)	$383,000	-	$193,000
Highest offered base salary (3)	$500,000	-	$380,000
Lowest offered base salary (3)	$210,000	-	$170,000
SK&A count of physicians (4)	17,303	38,132	24,904

Salary Guidelines	Endocrinologists	Family Medicine Physicians	Gastroenterologists
Median salary (1)	$221,400	$219.362	$435,120
Median work RVUs(1)	4,393	4,890	7,992
Median gross charges (1)	$637,191	$699,060	$1,801,861
Mean salary for men (2)	-	$184,000	$349,000
Mean salary for women (2)	–	$157,000	$308,000
Highest-paying region (2)	-	North Central ($186,000)	Northwest ($498,000)
Lowest-paying region (2)	–	Northwest ($162,000)	Mid-Atlantic ($311,000) 000)
Hospital-employed salary (2)	–	$204,000	$264,000
Multispecialty group practice salary (2)	-	$191,000	$421,000
Highest offered base salary (3)	$380,000	$300,000	$550,000
Lowest offered base salary (3)	$180,000	$120,000	$300,000
SK&A count of physicians (4)	6,578	121,528	19,682

Salary Guidelines	General surgeons	Hematologists/ Oncologists	Hospitalists
Median salary (1)	$370,024	$348,157	$236,500
Median work RVUs(1)	7,026	6,159	4,021
Median gross charges (1)	$1,347,674	$697,249	$437,100

Mean salary for men (2)	$290,000	$293,000	335000*'
Mean salary for women (2)	$225,000	$240,000	275000"
Highest-paying region (2)	North Central ($340,000)	Southwest ($347,000)	Southern ($247,000)**
Lowest-paying region (2)	Northwest ($258,000)	Northeast ($230,000)	Eastern ($212,000)"
Hospital-employed salary (2)	$262,000	$227,000	221928"
Multispecialty group practice salary (2)	$338,000	$356,000	-
Highest offered base salary (2)	$450.000	$450,000	$305,000
Lowest offered base salary (3)	$220,000	$210,000	$160,000
SK&A count of physicians (4)	21,507	16,012	N/An

Salary Guidelines	Internal Medicine	Neurologists	Obstetricians/ Gynecologists
Median salary (1)	$224,417	$249,250	$303,350
Median work RVUs(1)	4,717	4,717	6,476
Median gross charges (1)	$693,162	$754,216	$1,186,319
Mean salary for men (2)	$195,000	$227.000	$253,000
Mean salary for women (2)	$165,000	$189,000	$221,000
Highest-paying region (2)	South Central ($21 0,000)	South Central ($250,000)	South Central ($250,000)

Lowest-paying region (2)	Northeast ($168,000)	Mid-Atlantic ($194,000)	Mid-Atlantic ($194,000)
Hospital-employed salary (2)	$192,000	$199,000	$216,000
Multispecialty group practice salary (2)	$203,000	$226,000	$252.000
Highest offered base salary (3)	$345,000	$420,000	$440,000
Lowest offered base salary (3)	$150,000	$160,000	$180,000
SK&A count of physicians (4)	82,429	16,712	42,714

Salary Guidelines	Ophthalmologists	Orthopedic Surgeons	Otolaryngologists
Median salary (1)	$371,987	$515759	$374,387
Median work RVUs(1)	8,649	8,026	6,891
Median gross charges (1)	$1,665,174	$1.916,904	$1,532,766
Mean salary for men (2)	$294,000	$403,000	-
Mean salary for women (2)	$220,000	$422,000	-
Highest-paying region (2)	North Central ($352,000)	Northwest ($652,000}	-
Lowest-paying region (2)	South Central ($230,000)	Mid-Atlantic ($248,000)	-
Hospital-employed salary (2)	$205,000	$396,000	-
Multispecialty group practice salary (2^j	$340,000	$422,000	_

Highest offered base salary (3)	$450,000	$750,000	$530,000
Lowest offered base salary (3)	$145,000	$400,000	$300,000
SK&A count of physicians (4)	27,366	40,302	14,125

Salary Guidelines	Pediatricians	Pulmonologists	Urologists
Median salary (1)	$220,644	$304,900	$415,598
Median work RVUs(1)	5.111	6,057	7,456
Median gross charges (1)	$808,399	$929,103	$1,850,017
Mean salary for men (2)	$190,000	$219,000	$344,000
Mean salary for women (2)	$156,000	$271.000	$303,000
Highest-paying region (2)	Great Lakes ($182,000)	West ($296,000)	Great Lakes ($433,000)
Lowest-paying region (2)	North East ($165,000)	Southwest ($2 10,000)	Mid-Atlantic ($309,000)
Hospital-employed salary (2)	$162,000	$210,000	$328,000
Multispecialty group practice salary (2)	$188,000	$303.000	$412.000
Highest offered base salary (3)	$220,000	$415,000	$650,000
Lowest offered base salary (3)	S 1 50 DUO	$180,000	$330,000
SK&A count of physicians (4)	53,187	6,145	15,498

Footnotes

Information found in the AMGA Medical Group Compensation and Financial Survey, a 2012 report based on 2011 data.

Information found in Medscape's 2013 Physician Compensation Report.

Information found in Merritt Hawkins' 2013 Review of Physician Recruiting Incentives.

Information on physician count comes from SK&A, a Cegedim Company's 2013 database of office-based physicians.

* Highest and lowest offered salaries do not include bonuses."2012 Data

INDEX

A

B

C

D

E

F

H

J

K

L

M

O

P

S

W

www.ingramcontent.com/pod-product-compliance
Lightning Source LLC
Chambersburg PA
CBHW020726180526
45163CB00001B/132
9781499083392